Quick Review in Clinical Periodontics

Quick Review in Clinical Periodontics

Swati Gupta MDS (Periodontics)
SRF, Department of Pharmaceutics and
Nanotechnology (DST)
Panjab University
Chandigarh, India

Sumit Gupta BDS
Clinical Consultant
Chandigarh, India

CBS

CBS Publishers & Distributors Pvt Ltd

New Delhi • Bengaluru • Chennai • Kochi • Kolkata • Mumbai
Hyderabad • Jharkhand • Nagpur • Patna • Pune • Uttarakhand

Disclaimer

Science and technology are constantly changing fields. New research and experience broaden the scope of information and knowledge. The authors have tried their best in giving information available to them while preparing the material for this book. Although all efforts have been made to ensure optimum accuracy of the material, yet it is quite possible some errors might have been left uncorrected. The publisher, the printer and the authors will not be held responsible for any inadvertent errors or inaccuracies.

Quick Review in
Clinical Periodontics

ISBN: 978-93-86478-65-8

First Edition: 2017

Published by Satish Kumar Jain and produced by Varun Jain for

CBS Publishers & Distributors Pvt Ltd

4819/XI Prahlad Street, 24 Ansari Road, Daryaganj, New Delhi 110 002, India.

Ph: 23289259, 23266861, 23266867 Website: www.cbspd.com

Fax: 011-23243014 e-mail: delhi@cbspd.com; cbspubs@airtelmail.in.

Corporate Office: 204 FIE, Industrial Area, Patparganj, Delhi 110 092

Ph: 4934 4934 Fax: 4934 4935 e-mail: publishing@cbspd.com; publicity@cbspd.com

Branches

- **Bengaluru:** Seema House 2975, 17th Cross, K.R. Road, Banasankari 2nd Stage, Bengaluru 560 070, Karnataka
  Ph: +91-80-26771678/79 Fax: +91-80-26771680 e-mail: bangalore@cbspd.com
- **Chennai:** 7, Subbaraya Street, Shenoy Nagar, Chennai 600 030, Tamil Nadu
  Ph: +91-44-26680620, 26681266 Fax: +91-44-42032115 e-mail: chennai@cbspd.com
- **Kochi:** Ashana House, No. 39/1904, AM Thomas Road, Valanjambalam, Ernakulam 682 016, Kochi, Kerala
  Ph: +91-484-4059061-65 Fax: +91-484-4059065 e-mail: kochi@cbspd.com
- **Kolkata:** 6/B, Ground Floor, Rameswar Shaw Road, Kolkata-700 014, West Bengal
  Ph: +91-33-22891126, 22891127, 22891128 e-mail: kolkata@cbspd.com
- **Mumbai:** 83-C, Dr E Moses Road, Worli, Mumbai-400018, Maharashtra
  Ph: +91-22-24902340/41 Fax: +91-22-24902342 e-mail: mumbai@cbspd.com

Representatives

- **Hyderabad** 0-9885175004 • **Jharkhand** 0-9811541605 • **Nagpur** 0-9021734563
- **Patna** 0-9334159340 • **Pune** 0-9623451994 • **Uttarakhand** 0-9716462459

Printed at Nutech Print Services, Faridabad, India

Foreword

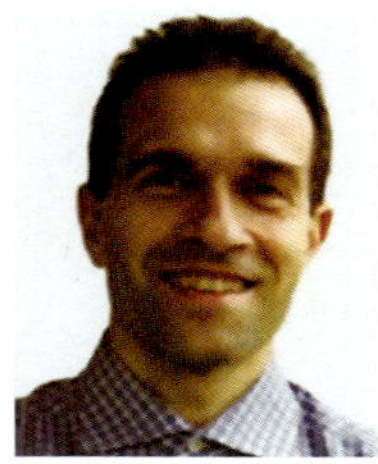

Mentoring means teaching others not just technical or scientific knowledge, but especially the tips and tricks acquired with years of experience, that may help young practitioners to perform their jobs properly without making common mistakes already made by others. Therefore, the mentor is usually seen as a middle- or old-aged person, usually the leader of a team, who is available to sharing his/her long term experience. In spite of the young age of the author, this book is written with the spirit of a mentor that aims at providing the best possible advice to the readers, supposedly undergraduate and young postgraduate students, but indeed it can be helpful also to the less young practitioners in periodontics field.

In fact, the book is written with a fluent language, very practical and easy to understand. The different topics are described in a concise way without leaving out anything essential, and are illustrated with clear pictures, sketches and detailed description of clinical cases. Furthermore, many inserts are present, with insights on specific topics, clinical notes and practical procedures, described step-by-step. Also, they synthesize the main advices and practical guidelines, useful to any practitioner in order to perform correct diagnosis and provide the most appropriate treatment in clinical periodontics according to an effective integration between evidence-based medicine directions and personal experience.

Virtually all aspects of the clinical periodontology field are covered, with frequent reference to the most eminent scientific literature and to worldwide approved classifications and guidelines. The book is ideal for clinicians who look for a practical manual, a reference to consult in case of doubts regarding differential diagnosis and alternative treatments.

Concluding, I enjoyed reading this book and recommend it to all undergraduate and postgraduate students as well as professionals, as a valuable companion to more famous and eminent textbooks of periodontology, with the advantage of an easier and practice-oriented language, that may be appreciated at first sight.

Prof Massimo Del Fabbro
Università degli Studi di Milano
Dipartimento di Scienze Biomediche,
Chirurgiche e Odontoiatriche
Istituto Ortopedico Galeazzi IRCCS
Via Riccardo Galeazzi 4
20161 Milano
Italy

Preface

Periodontology is a vast and diversified subject with complexities of various aspects of dental problems including surgeries. Students both at undergraduate and postgraduate level experience enormous difficulties and confusion in understanding the take away points for exams and for applying theoretical knowledge to clinical practice. Time and again students struggle to master the judgment and skills required to make a clinical decision. Hence, the thought of writing this book occurred to me. This is not a textbook *per se* but contains the tips and toes of the surgical/theoretical aspects of surgical topics in its first part. This clinically oriented text provides the essential information required to diagnose periodontal tissues in health and disease, and deliver effective treatment. Written in a user-friendly language and style, we have tried to encompass all the updated classification, indices and surgical treatments with color images. This textbook is a valuable resource not only for students but also dental practitioners.

A thorough reading and understanding of the information contained in this book is quite beneficial to understand the veracities of clinical pathologies. It would be equally helpful for general dental practitioners as well as those newly starting in secondary care. Students would find this book helpful as it contains easy to go through concepts required to prepare before any theory examination. Important chair-side points, *viva voce* as well as clinical notes have been highlighted separately. This book will act as a ready reckoner for the students to provide them important inputs for MCQs and theory exams, easy to comprehend and memorize within a short time. However, students are required to go through standard textbooks for a detailed knowledge of the subject. Lindhe, Carranza, Polson, Perio 2000, Gickmann are a few books from which important points have been summarized for a better understanding of the subject.

Swati Gupta
Sumit Gupta

Acknowledgements

First and the foremost, I would like to thank the positive energy 'the Supreme' who has made this possible!

This book is for the strivers, young dentists who work against the odds, polish their skills and theory with clinical practice. I sincerely hope that my book would serve as a constant reminder to the young readers to never stop trying!

I am highly indebted to the publishers (CBSPD) and their entire team for accepting and producing my work magnificently in the bookform.

I would like to thank Dr Pratibha PK, Professor and Head, Department of Periodontics, Manipal University, for being my mentor and a guiding beacon throughout. I am extremely grateful to Dr KM Bhat, Dr GS Bhat, Dr Betsy Thomas and Dr Kanishk Gupta for their mentoring. A big thanks to all the students whose queries and problems made me think about writing this book.

I extend my deepest and heartfelt gratitude to my parents Brijesh Gupta and K K Gupta for their round the clock constant support, encouragement and guidance. The thought of writing would not have become a reality, if not the inspiring words of my brother Dr Sumit Gupta (coauthor) and my sisters Dr Richa Gupta and Minoti Gupta. This book is a culmination of hardwork and cooperation of my family members.

My dearest friends and critics Dr Sanjana Ravi Kumar and Dr Hrishi TS have played a significant role in proofreading and improving the book with their innovative ideas.

I dedicate this book to my nieces—Zufisha and Aahana!

Swati Gupta

Contents

1 Gingiva

The gingiva is that part of oral mucosa (masticatory mucosa) that covers the alveolar process of the jaws and surrounds the necks of the teeth.

Gingiva achieves its final shape and texture in conjunction with eruption of teeth.

Gingiva is divided anatomically into (Fig. 1.1a and b):

1. Marginal/unattached/free gingiva
2. Attached gingiva (AG)
3. Interdental areas

1. The free gingiva is coral pink, has a dull surface and firm consistency. After complete tooth eruption, the free gingival margin is located on the enamel surface approximately 1.52 mm coronal to the cementoenamel junction.
2. The attached gingiva is demarcated by the free gingival groove (GG). A free gingival groove is only present in about 30–40% of adults.
3. Along the vestibular and lingual aspects of the alveolar ridge, a mucogingival junction (MJ) demarcates the normally light pink, firmly bound gingiva from the dark-red, movable alveolar mucosa or the floor of the mouth mucosa.

Note: *There is no mucogingival line in palate. Hard palate and alveolar process are covered by same type of masticatory mucosa* (Fig. 1.2).

Width of Attached Gingiva

Incisor region: 3.5–4.5 mm (maxilla), 3.3–3.9 mm in mandible
Posterior region: 1.9 mm (maxilla), 1.8 mm (mandible)

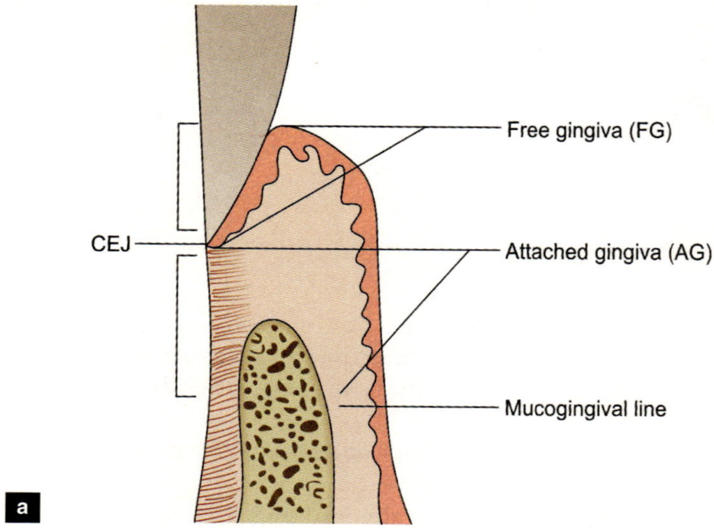

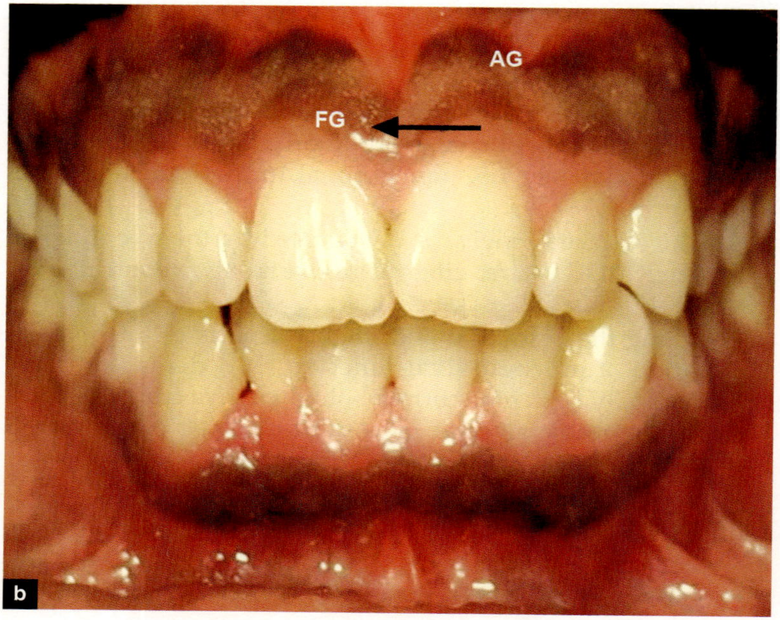

Fig. 1.1a and b: Clinically normal gingiva. The core of interdental papilla is formed by attached gingiva (marked in arrow)

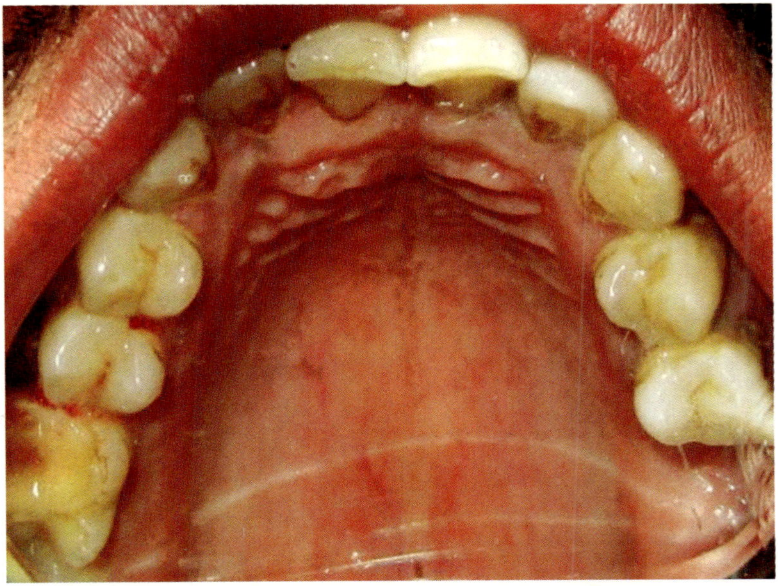

Fig. 1.2: Palatal masticatory mucosa. No mucogingival line in palate

Clinical Note

The mucogingival junction, particularly on the vestibular aspect, can be localized:

- *Functionally—by passive movement of the lips and cheek.*
- *Anatomically—by difference of color and surface characteristics such as stippling.*
- *Histochemically—by application of Schillers iodine solution to reveal the glycogen stored in the epithelium of the lining mucosa.*
- *LA test: Injection of local anesthesia will show the elevation in area of mucogingival junction.*
- *Roll test: To determine the attached gingival width insufficiency primarily.*

Correlation of Clinical and Macroscopic Features

1. *Color:* It varies with the thickness and degree of keratinization of epithelium, vascular supply and the pigment containing melanin cells.

   Melanin pigmentation is seen as early as 3 hours after birth.
2. *Size:* It is sum total of bulk of cellular and intercellular elements and the vascular supply. Gingival thickness ranges between

0.5 and 2.5 mm vestibularly and is inversely proportional to gingival height.

3. *Contour:* Depends on shape of teeth, alignment of teeth in the arch, location and size of area of proximal contact, dimensions of facial and lingual gingival embrasures. It can be scalloped, accentuated and flat.
   a. Scalloped on facial and lingual surfaces (Fig. 1.3).
   b. Accentuated contour—on teeth in labial version or with pronounced mesiodistal convexity (Fig. 1.4).
   c. Horizontal and thickened—on teeth inclined lingually.

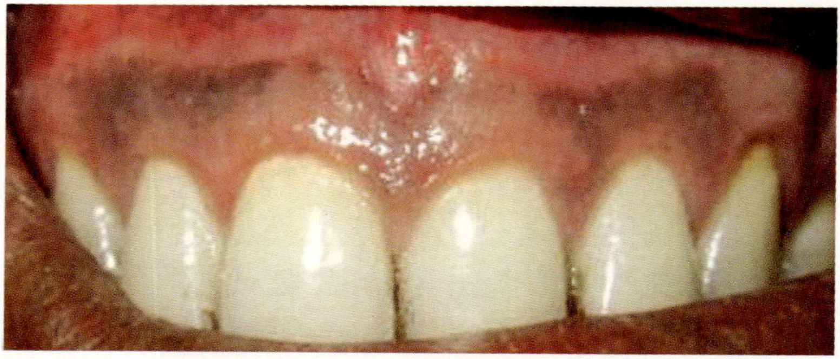

Fig. 1.3: Scalloped contour of gingiva with melanin pigmentation. Stippling can be seen in attached gingiva of maxillary central incisors

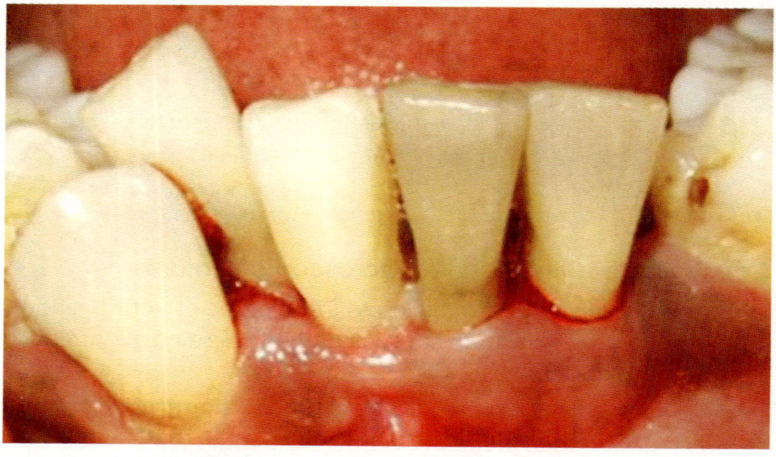

Fig. 1.4: Flat contour of gingiva in teeth in labial position

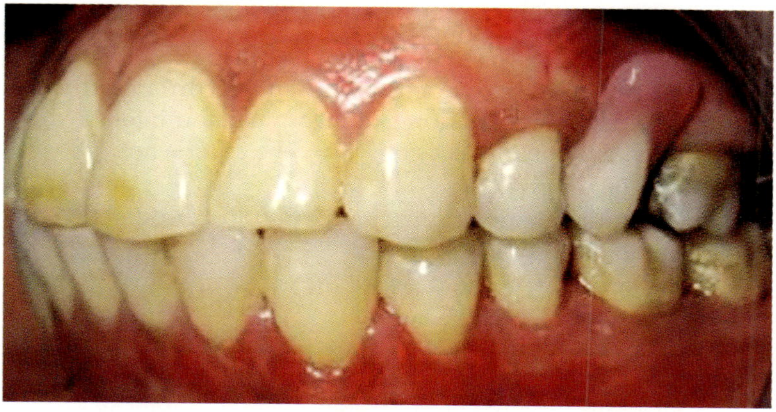

Fig. 1.5: Shape of interdental papilla. (a) Pyramidal in anterior; (b) Flattened in posterior

4. *Shape:* It is governed by contour of proximal tooth surface and location of gingival embrasure (Fig. 1.5).
   a. Pyramidal interdental papilla—anterior
   b. Flattened molar region
5. *Consistency:* Firm and resilient in healthy gingiva. This is attributed to collagenous nature of lamina propria (connective tissue layer) and its contiguity with mucoperiosteum of bone.
6. *Surface texture:* Stippled (orange peel) is seen in healthy gingiva.
   a. Stippling is seen in attached gingiva and core of interdental papilla.
   b. Appears at 5 years of age and disappears in old age.
   c. It is a form of adaptive specialization or reinforcement of function. Loss of stippling is a common sign of gingival disease.

Note: *Various theories for the appearance of stippling have been proposed. Most accepted is that it is produced by the projection of papillary layer into the elevations and depressions of epithelium of gingival surface.*

7. *Position:* Level at which gingival margin is attached to the tooth surface.

Gingival Index (GI)

The gingival index (Loe and Silness, 1963) was created for the assessment of the gingival condition and records qualitative changes in the gingiva. It scores the marginal and interproximal tissues separately on the basis of 0 to 3. The criteria are:

0 = Normal gingiva;

1 = Mild inflammation slight change in color and slight edema but no bleeding on probing;

2 = Moderate inflammation redness, edema and glazing, bleeding on probing;

3 = Severe inflammation marked redness and edema, ulceration with tendency to spontaneous bleeding.

The bleeding is assessed by probing gently along the wall of soft tissue of the gingival sulcus. The scores of the four areas of the tooth can be summed and divided by four to give the GI for the tooth. The GI of the individual can be obtained by adding the values of each tooth and dividing by the number of teeth examined. The gingival index may be scored for all surfaces of all or selected teeth or for selected areas of all or selected teeth. The GI may be used for the assessment of prevalence and severity of gingivitis in populations, groups and individuals.

A score from

0.1–1.0 = mild inflammation;

1.0–2.0 = moderate inflammation, and

2.1–3.0 = signifies severe inflammation.

The GI has been used frequently in clinical trials of therapeutic agents. The sensitivity and reproducibility is good.

Sulcus Bleeding Index (SBI)

An early sign of gingivitis is bleeding on probing, and in 1971; Muhlemann and Son described the sulcus bleeding index (SBI). The criteria for scoring are as follows:

Score 0: Healthy looking papillary and marginal gingiva no bleeding on probing

Score 1: Healthy looking gingiva, bleeding on probing;

Score 2: Bleeding on probing, change in color, no edema;

Score 3: Bleeding on probing, change in color, slight edema;

Score 4: Bleeding on probing, change in color, obvious edema;

Score 5: Spontaneous bleeding, change in color, marked edema

Four gingival units are scored systematically for each tooth: the labial and lingual marginal gingival (M units) and the mesial and distal papillary gingival (P units). Scores for these units are added and divided by four. Adding the scores of the undivided teeth and dividing them by the number of teeth can determine the sulcus bleeding index.

Papillary Bleeding Index (PBI)

The papillary bleeding index was first introduced by Saxer and Muhlemann (1975), as cited by Muhlemann (1977). This index permits both immediate evaluation of the patient's gingival condition and his motivation, based upon the actual bleeding tendency of the gingival papillae. A periodontal probe is inserted into the gingival sulcus at the base of the papilla on the mesial aspect, and then moved coronally to the papilla tip. This is repeated on the distal aspect of the papilla. The intensity of any bleeding is recorded as:

Score 0: No bleeding;
Score 1: A single discreet bleeding point;
Score 2: Several isolated bleeding points or a single line of blood appears;
Score 3: The interdental triangle fills with blood shortly after probing;
Score 4: Profuse bleeding occurs after probing; blood flows immediately into the marginal sulcus.

Eastman Interdental Bleeding Index (EIBI)

Caton and Polson (1985) developed the Eastman interdental bleeding (EIB) index. A wooden interdental cleaner is inserted between the teeth from the facial aspect, depressing the interdental tissues 1 to 2 mm. This is repeated four times and the presence or absence of bleeding within 15 sec is recorded.

Gingival Bleeding Index (GBI)

In 1974, Carter and Barnes introduced a gingival bleeding index, which records the presence or absence of gingival inflammation after passing unwaxed dental floss into the proximal sulcus. It is readily available, disposable, and can be used by the instructed patient for self-evaluation. The mouth is divided into six segments and flossed in the following order—upper right, upper anterior, upper left, lower left, lower anterior and lower right.

Bleeding is generally immediately evident in the area or on the floss; however, 30 sec is allowed for reinspection of each segment. If copious hemorrhage occurs, the patient may be allowed to rinse in between segments. Bleeding is recorded as present or absent. For each patient, a gingival bleeding score is obtained by noting the total units of bleeding and the total susceptible areas at risk.

Author's Note

An understanding of normal clinical features of gingiva—color, size, contour, shape, consistency, surface texture, and position should be done in a sequential order at the first appointment to determine the gingival status of the patient.

a. *Color determination will be helpful in determining underlying diseases, ethnicity and habits of the patient.*
b. *Alteration in size is a common feature of gingival disease.*
c. *Contour determines the thickness of gingival biotype and varies with alignment of teeth in the arch.*
d. *Consistency of diseased gingiva is soft and leathery as compared to firm and resilient in healthy.*
e. *Change in position of gingiva could be physiological as well as pathological and should be differentiated with a thorough examination.*

These changes have been discussed in detail in next chapter.

2 Gingivitis

Gingivitis is defined by the inflammation of the gingiva.

Stages of gingivitis by Page and Schroeder, 1976 are described in Table 2.1.

Table 2.1: Stages of gingivitis (Page and Schroeder, 1976)

Stage and time in days	*Histological findings*			*Clinical findings*
Stage I. Initial lesion (2–4 days)	Dilation of arterioles, capillaries and venules. Increased permeability. Perivascular loss of collagen occurs.	Junctional and sulcular epithelia are infiltrated by PMNs	PMNs appear due to diapedesis emigration in the dento-gingival vasculature	GCF flow is increased
Stage II. Early lesion (4–7 days)	Increase in vascular proliferation Loss of collagen around the inflammatory infiltrate.	Proliferation of rete-pegs 70% of collagen destruction	Lymphocytes, PMNs and a few plasma cells. Fibroblasts in the process of degeneration.	Marked redness bleeding on probing is evident
Stage III. Established lesion (14–21 days)	Blood vessel stasis occurs (anoxemia)—bluish hue on reddened gingiva. Extravasation of erythrocytes	Further rete-peg proliferation Junctional epithelium is substituted by pocket epithelium,	Plasma and B cell domination. Predominantly IgG1 and IgG3.	Change in color, size, texure, etc. It is of two types: 1. Stable—does not progress

(*Contd.*)

Table 2.1: Stages of gingivitis (Page and Schroeder, 1976) *(Contd.)*

Stage and time in days	*Histological findings*			*Clinical findings*
		which is more permeable to noxious due to ulcerations		2. Active: Converts to destructive lesions
Stage IV. Advanced lesion/ phase of periodontal breakdown	Increased dilatation and permeability	Deeper extension into connective tissue with severe loss of collagen. Apical migration along the root from the CEJ. Beginning of alveolar bone loss	Plasma cells are dominant in connective tissue. *Neutrophils continue dominant in junctional epithelium*	Resistance to probing

Note: *A. Gingivitis is not always due to accumulation of plaque on the tooth surface. It can be due to several causes, such as specific bacterial, viral or fungal infection without an associated plaque related gingival inflammatory reaction.*

Autoimmune causes, gingival lesions of genetic origin, allergies, and traumatic causes could be other factors.

B. The main fiber groups to be affected in Stage II gingivitis are circular and dentogingival fiber groups.

C. Advanced lesion—phase of periodontal breakdown. Gingivitis progresses to periodontitis only in susceptible patients.

The two earliest signs of gingival inflammation are:

1. Increased gingival crevicular fluid production rate
2. Bleeding from the gingival sulcus on gentle probing

Note: *Gingival bleeding on probing may not be a good diagnostic indicator for* clinical attachment loss but its absence is an excellent negative predictor of future attachment loss (Lang et al,1986).

Clinical Point

Probing to check bleeding should be done from posterior to anterior and the clinician should wait for 30 seconds for bleeding points to appear.

CLINICAL CHANGES IN GINGIVITIS

I. Abnormal gingival bleeding: The most common cause of abnormal gingival bleeding on probing is chronic inflammation. The color in chronic inflammation is red or bluish red because of vascular proliferation and reduction of keratinization.

a. Spontaneous bleeding or bleeding on slight provocation can occur in ANUG.
b. Hemorrhagic disorders: Vascular abnormalities, platelet disorders, hypoprothrombinemia, other coagulation defects, deficient platelet thromboplastic factor and multiple myeloma.
c. Hormonal replacement therapy, oral contraceptives, pregnancy, and the menstrual cycle affect gingival bleeding.

II. Changes in color

a. Endogenous oral melanin pigmentation: It can be caused by melanin, bilirubin or deposition of iron in hemochromatosis.
b. Exogenous factors include atmospheric irritants such as coal, metal dust, lead, mercury, bismuth, amalgam tattoo.
c. Diseases that increase melanin pigmentation: Addison's disease, Peutz-Jeghers syndrome, Albright's syndrome and Von Recklinghausen's syndrome.

III. Effects of toothbrushing: It has various effects on the consistency of gingiva such as promoting keratinization of the oral epithelium, enhancing capillary gingival circulation and thickening of alveolar bone.

Clinical Note

- *Traumatic ulcerative gingival lesion: Abrasiveness of dentifrice, strong brushing force, and horizontal movement of the toothbrush contribute to the gingival injury. Characteristics of these lesions are: Extremely good oral hygiene, cervical tooth abrasion, and unaffected tops of the interdental papillae at the site of injury (Fig. 2.1).*
- *Dental flossing may also cause gingival ulceration and inflammation primarily affecting the top of the interdental papillae.*
- *Gingivitis artefacta: Self-inflicted physical injury to the gingival tissues can occur due to habits like nail biting.*

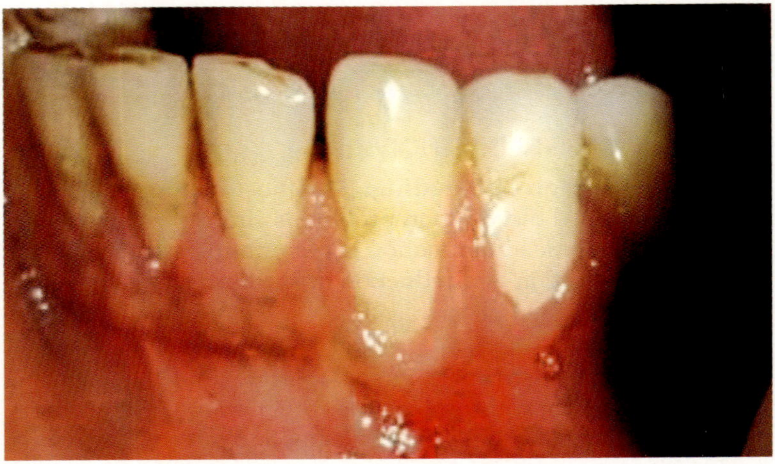

Fig. 2.1: Example of traumatic gingival lesion due to dentifrices. Note the cervical abrasions on facial surface and unaffected interdental papilla

IV. Changes in position of gingiva

a. Actual position: It is determined by the level of coronal end of the epithelial attachment on tooth.
b. Apparent position: It indicates the level of the crest of gingival margin.

Gingival recession is not physiological phenomenon and increases with age.

Clinical Point

Gingival recession is a condition whereas mucogingival problems are a diagnosis.

Gingival recession can result in: Caries, hypersensitivity, hyperemic pulp, interproximal recession craters, and plaque accumulation.

V. Changes in gingival contour

a. Stillman's clefts: Narrow triangular shaped gingival recession (Fig. 2.2).
b. McCall's festoons: Roll thickened band of gingiva in anteriors.

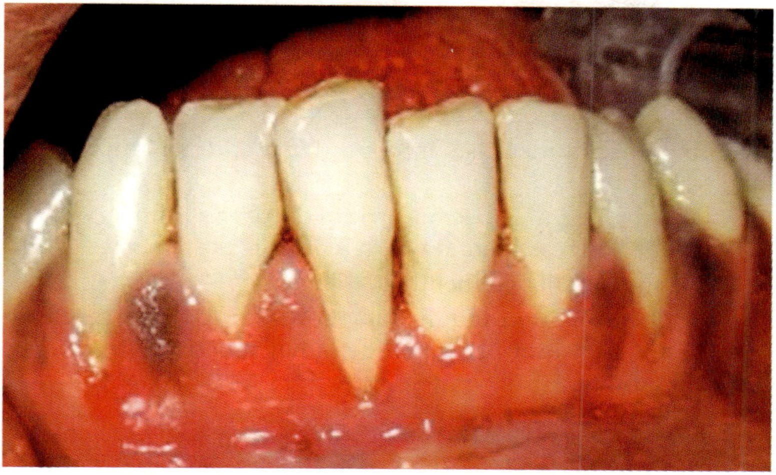

Fig. 2.2: Stillman's cleft in lower anteriors

Clinical Point

Stillman's clefts and the McCall's festoons are not associated with trauma from occlusion. These are due to chronic inflammation.

VI. Changes in surface texture of gingiva: Stippling is localized to attached gingiva (subpapillary area), may extend to interdental papilla. (*Core of interdental papilla is formed by* attached gingiva.)

Smooth texture in atrophic gingivitis, nodular surface in drug induced enlargements.

VII. Change in size of gingiva: Chronic gingival enlargement

1. Chronic inflammatory, drug induced
2. *According to location and distribution:* Localized (limited to gingiva of tooth or group of teeth), generalized (involving gingival throughout the mouth)
3. *Marginal:* Involving marginal gingiva
   Papillary: Confined to interdental papilla
   Diffuse: Confined to marginal, attached gingiva and interdental papilla.

Changes in Periodontium of Deciduous Dentition

1. No interdental col formation: Interdental papilla is well keratinized and saddle-shaped, referred to as interdental saddle.

2. Stippling appears around after 3–5 years of age and diminishes in old age.
3. Gingival sulcus is shallower than permanent dentition with a mean depth of 2.1 ±0.2 mm.
4. Probing depth increases in depth from anterior to posterior (1 to 2 mm).
5. Attached gingiva (3 to 6 mm) width decreases from anterior to posterior whereas lingual width increases posteriorly.
6. Thicker junctional epithelium
7. R/F: Crest of interdental bony septa is flat and septa lie within 1 to 2 mm of cementoenamel junction. Prominent lamina dura.

Note: *The most prevalent type of gingival disease in children is chronic marginal gingivitis (does not progress to periodontitis as gingivitis in children is T lymphocyte dominated, a few B cells), also children have thicker junctional epithelium (less permeability to bacterial toxins).*

Eruption cyst: Refers to gingival bulge in lower incisors and 1st molar area.

Microorganisms in childhood gingivitis: *Actinomyces, Capnocytophaga, Leptotrichia, Selenomonas*.

The American Academy of Periodontology 1989 proposed the following classification of periodontitis:

I. Adult periodontitis
II. Early-onset periodontitis
   A. Prepubertal periodontitis
      1. Generalized
      2. Localized
   B. Juvenile periodontitis
      1. Generalized
      2. Localized
   C. Rapidly progressive periodontitis
III. Periodontitis associated with systemic disease
IV. Necrotizing ulcerative periodontitis
V. Refractory periodontitis.

Note: *Acute lymphocytic leukemia is most common in children.*

Influences of Systemic Diseases on Periodontitis in Children and Adolescents

Systemic disorders associated with periodontitis in children are: Neutropenia, Chédiak-Higashi syndrome, leukocyte adhesion deficiency syndrome, Papillon-Lefevre syndrome, Down's syndrome, hypophosphatasia, Ehlers-Danlos syndrome, acquired immune deficiency syndrome.

Classification of Periodontal Diseases and Conditions (Carranza 12th ed)

I. **Gingival diseases:** Plaque-induced gingival diseases, non-plaque-induced gingival diseases
II. **Chronic periodontitis:** Localized, generalized
III. **Aggressive periodontitis:** Localized, generalized
IV. **Periodontitis as a manifestation of systemic diseases**
   A. *Necrotizing periodontal diseases:* Necrotizing ulcerative gingivitis, necrotizing ulcerative periodontitis
   B. *Abscesses of the periodontium:* Gingival abscess, periodontal abscess, pericoronal abscess
   C. *Periodontitis associated with endodontic lesions:* Endodontic-periodontal lesion, periodontal-endodontic lesion, combined lesion
V. **Developmental or acquired deformities and conditions:**
   1. Localized tooth-related factors that predispose to plaque-induced gingival diseases or periodontitis
   2. Mucogingival deformities and conditions around teeth
   3. Mucogingival deformities and conditions on edentulous ridge
   4. Occlusal trauma

Classification of Gingival Diseases (Carranza 12th ed)

I. Plaque-induced gingival diseases
II. Non-plaque-induced gingival diseases

Plaque-induced gingival diseases: These occur on a periodontium with no attachment loss or on a periodontium with attachment loss that is stable and nonprogressing.

I. Gingivitis associated with dental plaque only:
   A. With local contributing factors
   B. Without local contributing factors

II. Gingival diseases modified by systemic factors:
   A. Associated with endocrine system:
      1. Puberty-associated gingivitis
      2. Menstrual cycle-associate gingivitis
      3. Pregnancy-associated gingivitis, pyogenic granuloma
      4. Diabetes mellitus-associated gingivitis
   B. Associated with blood dyscrasias
      1. Leukemia-associated gingivitis
      2. Others

III. Gingival disease modified by medications: Drug influenced gingival diseases
      1. Drug influenced gingival enlargements
      2. Drug influenced gingivitis—oral contraceptive-induced gingivitis, other

IV. Gingival diseases modified by malnutrition: Ascorbic acid deficiency gingivitis, other

Non-plaque-induced gingival lesions

I. Gingival diseases of specific bacterial origin: *Neisseria gonorrhoeae, T. pallidum, Streptococcus aureus*, others

II. Gingival diseases of viral origin
   A. Herpes virus infections: Primary herpetic gingivostomatitis, Recurrent oral herpes, varicella zoster
   B. Others

III. Gingival diseases of fungal origin:
   A. Candida species infections: Generalized gingival candidiasis
   B. Linear gingival erythema
   C. Histoplasmosis
   D. Other

IV. Gingival lesions of genetic origin:
   A. Hereditary gingival fibromatosis
   B. Others

V. Gingival manifestations of systemic diseases:
   A. Mucocutaneous lesions: Lichen planus, pemphigoid, pemphigus vulgaris, erythema multiforme, lupus erythematosus, others
   B. Allergic reactions:
      1. Due to restorative materials: Mercury, nickel, acrylic, other

2. Reactions attributable to: Toothpastes or dentifrices, mouthrinses or mouthwashes, chewing gum additives, foods and additives
3. Others

VI. **Traumatic lesions** (iatrogenic, accidental): Chemical injury, physical injury, thermal injury

VII. Foreign body reactions

VIII. Not otherwise specified

Classification of Periodontal Diseases (1999)

Periodontitis has been classified into three major types based on clinical, histological, radiographic and laboratory characteristics.

I. Chronic periodontitis

II. Aggressive periodontitis

III. Periodontitis as a manifestation of systemic diseases

I. **Chronic periodontitis:** Characteristics of chronic periodontitis patients are:

1. Prevalent in adults but occur in children
2. **Amount of destruction consistent with local factors**
3. **Associated with a variable microbial pattern**
4. Subgingival calculus frequently found
5. **Slow to moderate progression with periods of rapid progression**
6. **Possibly modified by or associated** with the following:
   a. Systemic diseases such as diabetes mellitus or HIV infection
   b. Local factors predisposing to periodontitis
   c. Environmental factors such as smoking and stress.

Chronic periodontitis is further subclassified into:

a. Localized form: <30% of sites involved

Clinical Note

Clinical attachment loss and clinical attachment level are synonyms.

For example: When clinical attachment level is 4 mm below CEJ, clinical attachment loss is 4 mm.

Clinical attachment level (CAL) measures the distance between the cementoenamel junction and the lowest point (pocket depth) using a periodontal probe.

b. Generalized form: <30% of sites involved
c. Slight: 1–2 mm of clinical attachment loss (CAL)
d. Moderate: 3–4 mm CAL
e. Severe: >5 mm of CAL

II. **Aggressive periodontitis:** Characteristics of aggressive periodontitis patients are:
1. Otherwise **clinically healthy patient**
2. **Rapid attachment loss and bone destruction**
3. **Amount of microbial deposits inconsistent with disease severity**
4. Familial aggregation of diseased individuals—A few characteristics which are common but not universal.
5. **Diseased sites infected with *Aggregatibacter actinomycetemcomitans*** (previously called *Actinobacillus actinomycetemcomitans*)
6. Abnormalities in phagocyte function
7. Hyperresponsive macrophages producing increased prostaglandin and interleukin
8. Self-arresting disease progression (in some cases)

Aggressive periodontitis has been further classified as given in Table 2.2.

Table 2.2: Classification of aggressive periodontitis

Localized form	*Generalized form*
1. Circumpubertal onset of disease	Usually affecting persons under <30 yrs of age
2. Localized first molar or incisor disease	Generalized proximal attachment loss
3. Proximal attachment loss on at least two permanent teeth, one of which is a first molar	Proximal attachment loss affecting at least three teeth other than first molar and incisors
4. Robust serum antibody response to infecting agents	Poor serum antibody response to infecting agents Pronounced episodic nature of periodontal destruction

Note: *The difference between chronic and aggressive periodontitis highlighted in bold points.*

III. **Periodontitis as a manifestation of systemic disease:** Periodontitis may be observed as a manifestation of systemic diseases:

1. *Hematologic disorders:* Acquired neutropenia, leukemia and others.
2. *Genetic disorders:* Familial and cyclic neutropenia, Down syndrome, glycogen storage diseases, Papillon-Lefevre syndrome, Cohen syndrome, hypophosphatasia, Chediak-Higashi syndrome, others.
3. Not otherwise specified.

Author's Note

a. *It is imperative to determine the stage of gingivitis as it helps the clinician in charting the treatment plan.*
b. *Clinicians should detect the early signs of gingivitis and carry out effective non-surgical therapy with continuous monitoring and recalls. Early stages can be reversed but require a longer time to heal.*
c. *Gingival size is an indicator of systemic diseases and side effects of various medications. Dental clinician could be the first to detect changes in the system by comprehensive gingival examination.*
d. *Gingival enlargements and their treatment are discussed in next chapter.*

3

Gingival Enlargements

Increase in size of the gingiva is called gingival enlargement or gingival overgrowth.

Classification

A. *According to etiologic factors and pathologic changes* (*Carranza 11th ed*):

I. Inflammatory enlargement: Acute (Fig. 3.1) and chronic (Fig. 3.2)

II. Drug-induced enlargement

III. Enlargements associated with systemic diseases or conditions

   a. *Conditioned enlargement:* Pregnancy, puberty, vitamin C deficiency, plasma cell gingivitis, nonspecific conditioned enlargement (pyogenic granuloma)

   b. *Systemic diseases causing gingival enlargement:* Leukemia, granulomatosis diseases (Wegener's granulomatosis, sarcoidosis)

IV. Neoplastic enlargement (gingival tumors):

   a. Benign tumors: Fibroma, papilloma, peripheral giant cell granuloma, gingival cysts, etc.

   b. Malignant tumors: Carcinoma, malignant melanoma

V. False enlargement

   a. Underlying osseous lesions: Tori, exostoses, Paget's disease, fibrous dysplasia, cherubism, central giant cell granuloma, ameloblastoma, osteoma, osteosarcoma.

   b. Underlying dental tissues: Developmental enlargement.

Methods to Assess Gingival Enlargement

Bokenkamp index (most commonly used)

Grade 0: No signs of gingival enlargement

Grade 1: Enlargement confined to interdental papilla

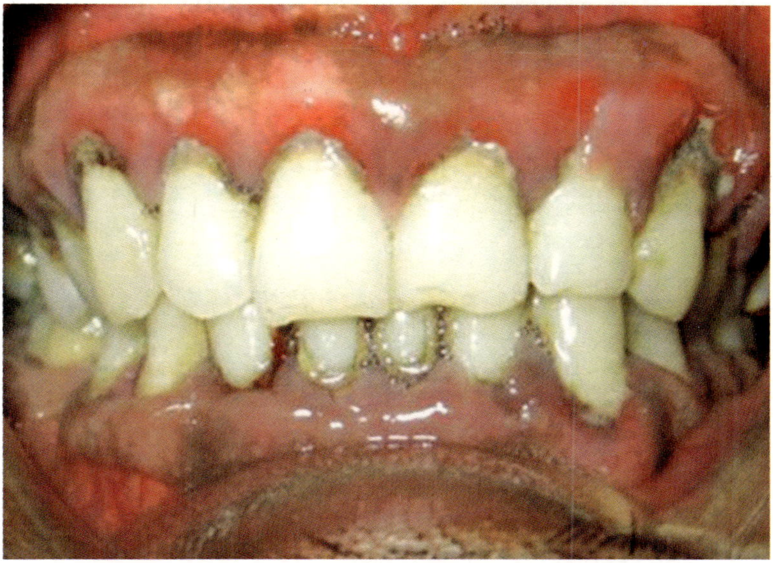

Fig. 3.1: Chronic inflammatory gingival enlargement

Grade 2: Enlargement involves papilla and marginal gingiva
Grade 3: Enlargement covers three quarters or more of the crown

Other indices: Harris and Ewalt index (1942), Cast method: by Ingle et al (1959), Aas index (1963), Angelopoulos and Goaz (1972), Miller and Dawn (1992), Seymour (1985) modified later by J. Miranda and Brunet (2001)

I. Acute Inflammatory Enlargement: Gingival Abscess, Periodontal (Lateral Abscess/Parietal Abscess)

1. Gingival abscess: Limited to marginal gingiva/interdental papilla.
2. Periodontal abscess (Fig. 3.2): Localized purulent inflammation in periodontal tissues. These are further classified according to location as:
   a. Abscess in the supporting tissues along the lateral aspect of the root: A sinus generally occurs in the bone.
   b. Abscess in the soft tissue wall of a deep periodontal pocket.

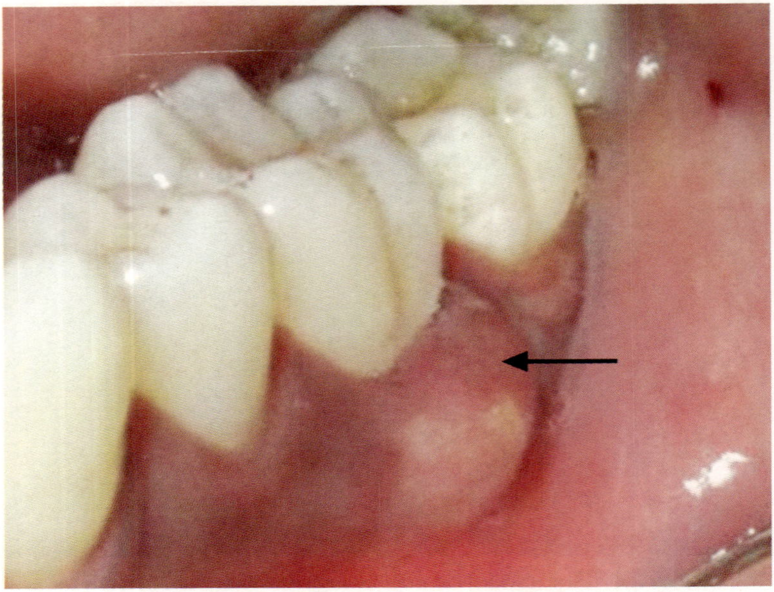

Fig. 3.2: Periodontal abscess in mandibular first molar

Periodontal abscess formation: The various routes that are possible have been mentioned:

1. Extension of inflammation from deep periodontal pocket into supporting periodontal tissues
2. Lateral extension of inflammation from the inner surface of pocket into connective tissue wall
3. Formation of pocket in the cul-de-sac around the root
4. Incomplete removal of calculus occluding the pocket orifice
5. After trauma to the root or perforation of the lateral wall of the root after endodontic therapy

Signs of Periodontal Abscess

1. *Acute abscess:* Mild to severe discomfort, periodontal pocket, tooth mobility, tooth elevation in socket, tenderness to percussion or biting, exudation, elevated temperature, regional lymphadenopathy.
2. *Chronic abscess:* No pain or dull pain, localized inflammatory lesion, slight tooth elevation, intermittent exudation, fistulous tract often associated with deep pocket.

Differential Diagnosis of Periodontal versus Periapical Abscess

Periodontal abscess	*Periapical abscess*
Pre-existing periodontal pocket	May have no periodontal pocket
Bone loss and furcation radiolucency	Not necessarily bone loss
Vital pulp	Nonvital pulp
Dull and localized pain	Severe pain and difficult to localize
Sensitive to percussion—may be absent	Sensitive to percussion

II. Drug-Induced Gingival Enlargement (DIGE)

Anticonvulsants, calcium channel blockers and immunosuppressant.

Drugs causing gingival overgrowth	
Anticonvulsants	Phenytoin, sodium valproate, phenobarbitone, primidone, ethosuximide
Immunosuppressant	Tacrolimus, cyclosporine
Calcium channel blockers	Nifedipine, felodipine, Amlodipine, verapamil, diltiazem

Common Characteristics of DIGE

1. All drug-induced enlargements show variation in interpatient and intrapatient pattern, i.e. genetic predisposition.
2. These enlargements are most commonly caused by phenytoin, cyclosporine A, or certain calcium channel blockers. They show predilection for anterior gingiva with the exception of phenobarbitone.
3. Higher prevalence in children and onset is within 3 months.
4. Enlargement first observed at the interdental papilla. Change in gingival contour leads to modification of gingival size. Gingival changes not necessarily are associated with bone loss.
5. Change in gingival color, increased gingival exudates, bleeding upon provocation.
6. Pronounced inflammatory response of gingiva in relation to the plaque present. Reductions in dental plaque can limit the severity of lesion.

A. *Anticonvulsants* (Fig. 3.3)

Etiology: Genetically determined gingival enlargement. Other causes relate to the metabolite of phenytoin, i.e. 5-(parahydroxyphenyl)-5-phenylhydantoin (5-p-HPPH). This metabolite stimulates:

1. Proliferation of fibroblast like cells,
2. Increased amounts of sulfated glycosaminoglycans (GAGs),

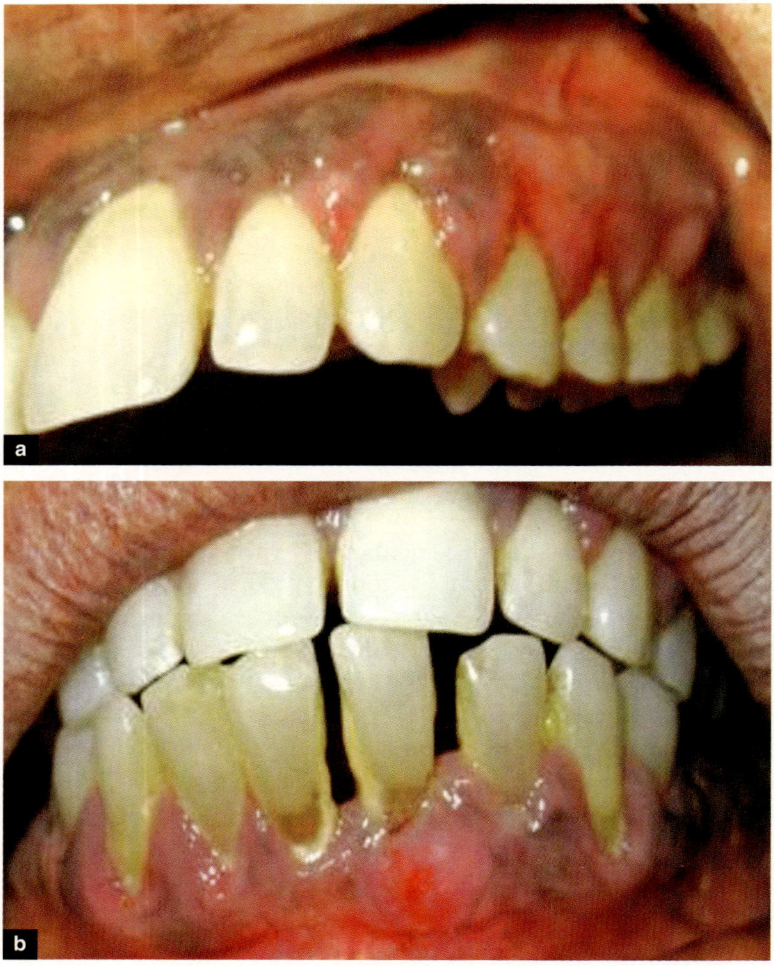

Fig. 3.3: A case of enlargement due to anticonvulsants in a female patient aged 45 years

3. Increased production of inactive fibroblast collagenase (decrease in collagen degradation),
4. Increase in tissue alkaline phosphatase activity.

B. *Immunosuppressants:* The enlargement is considered as hypersensitivity response by the body. It is characterized by:
1. Dosage greater than 500 mg/day causes gingival overgrowth.
2. Marked inflammatory changes. They bleed readily on probing and are generally more hyperemic.
3. Has **not been described in edentulous patients.**
4. Magnitude appears to be related to plasma concentration of the drug than patients periodontal status.

C. *Calcium channel blockers:* Most of the calcium channel blockers cause gingival enlargement except *Isradipine.*
1. Phenytoin and nifedipine—A stimulator for fibroblast growth
2. Calcium channel blocker induced enlargement **does not occur in edentulous areas**.
3. Adversely affects the secretory properties of gingival fibroblasts/collagenases, interferes with T cell activation and proliferation.

III. Idiopathic Gingival Enlargement

Also called gingivomatosis, elephantiasis, idiopathic fibromatosis, hereditary gingival hyperplasia, and congenital familial fibromatosis.
1. Affects attached gingiva as well as gingival margin and interdental papilla. **Involvement can be limited to either** jaw.
2. Avascular connective tissue.

Note: *Tuberous sclerosis is a triad of epilepsy, mental deficiency and cutaneous angiofibromas.*

IV. Conditioned Enlargements

These enlargements are magnification of an existing inflammation initiated by dental plaque. This is seen in pregnancy, puberty, vitamin C deficiency, non-specific conditioned enlargement (pyogenic granuloma).

A. *Enlargement in pregnancy:*
   1. It is histologically called angiogranuloma.

Note: *Estrogen has prominent effect on increase in vascular permeability, causing gingival edema leading to increased inflammatory response to dental plaque.*

2. Attributed to the increase in both progesterone (10 times) and estrogen (30 times).
3. Increases in 3rd month, becomes severe by 8th month and decreases during 9th month of pregnancy.
4. **Pronounced ease of bleeding** is a striking clinical feature.
5. Microorganism increased *Prevotella intermedia.*
6. More on interproximal surfaces than facial and lingual, raspberry like appearance.

B. *Enlargement in puberty* (Fig. 3.4): All the features associated with chronic inflammatory gingival disease. The characteristic features are:

1. Tendency to recur in the presence of relatively scant deposits.
2. The microorganism associated with pubertal gingivitis is *Capnocytophaga* spp.

C. *Enlargement in vitamin C deficiency:*

a. Acute deficiency of vitamin C does not cause gingival inflammation but does cause collagen degeneration and edema of gingival connective tissue.
b. Deficiency of vitamin C also called scurvy is characterized by impairment or cessation of osteoid formation, impaired osteoblastic function, defective formation and maintenance of collagen.

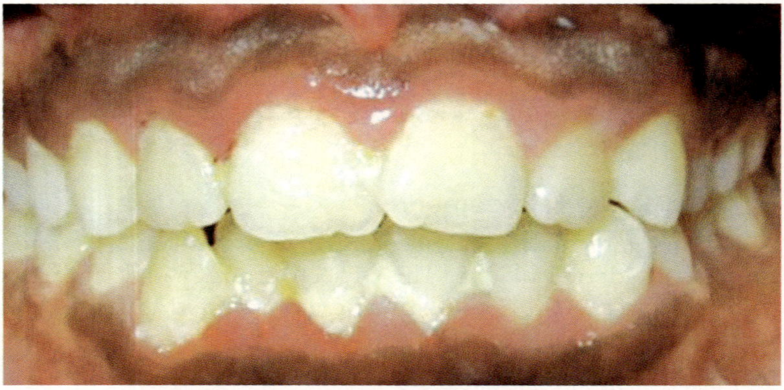

Fig. 3.4: Gingival enlargement in puberty

Note: *Role of ascorbic acid in periodontal disease has been hypothesized due to following reasons (Wolfe et al, 1980):*

a. Affected metabolism of collagen—affects the ability of tissues to regenerate and repair.

b. Interference with bone formation—osteoclastic resorption. Not associated with periodontal pocket formation.

c. Ascorbic acid deficiency increases the permeability to tritiated endotoxin and inulin. Epithelium barrier function is disrupted.

d. Impairs the bactericidal activity of leukocytes

e. Deficiency disrupts the integrity of periodontal microvasculature and vascular response to plaque.

f. Interference with the ecological equilibrium of bacteria in plaque and increases its pathogenicity.

Clinical manifestations: Hemorrhagic lesions into muscles of extremities, joints, nail beds, petechial hemorrhages, increased. susceptibility of infections, and sluggishness of blood flow, impaired wound healing.

Gingival manifestations: Bleeding swollen gingiva (boggy gums) characterized by bluish red, smooth shiny and friable surface, loosened teeth.

D. *Plasma cell gingivitis:* Considered to be allergic in origin. Related to components of chewing gum, dentifrices, and various diet components.

Clinical Note

Plasma cell gingivitis presents as localized lesion in oral aspect of attached gingiva. This is the main difference from plaque-induced gingivitis.

E. *Pyogenic granuloma* (*Fig. 3.5*): It is a tumor-like enlargement that is considered an exaggerated response to minor trauma. Its treatment is excision of the lesion along with elimination of irritating local factors.

V. Systemic Diseases that Cause Gingival Enlargement

Leukemic enlargement: Leukemia affects all cells of the body resulting in leucopenia, anemia, and thrombocytopenia. Leukemic cells, which are accumulation of immature blast cells, frequently

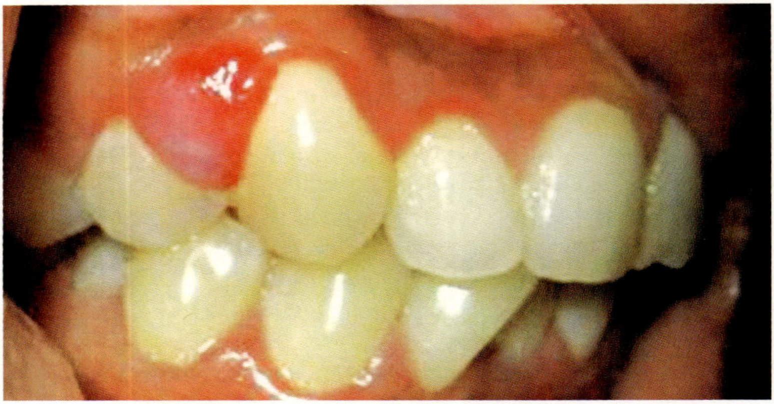

Fig. 3.5: Pyogenic granuloma in 19-year-old patient

infiltrate the gingiva, less frequently the alveolar bone. This enlargement is characterized by:

a. Leukemia enlargement does not occur in chronic leukemia and edentulous patients.
b. Bleeding gingiva is an early sign of leukemia (*occurs due to* secondary thrombocytopenia)
c. Marginal gingiva shows classical signs of ulceration, marginal necrosis with pseudomembrane formation.
d. Clinical manifestation: Gingiva is peculiar bluish red, sponge-like and friable, bleeds on the slightest provocation.

Note: *Leukemia cutis is an abnormal accumulation of leukemic cells in dermal and subcutaneous connective tissue.*

Aleukemic leukemia—patients have normal blood cell count while leukemic cells reside in bone marrow.

Enlargement of the bone is seen in Tori, exostosis, Paget's disease, fibrous dysplasia, cherubism, central giant cell granuloma, ameloblastoma, osteoma, and osteosarcoma.

Clinical Note

Difference between fibroma and epulis:

Epulis is a term used clinically to designate all discrete tumors and tumor like masses of gingiva.

Fibromas are slow growing tumors arising from gingival connective tissue and periodontal ligament.

Treatment of Gingival Enlargements

1. Plaque control is mandatory to control any kind of enlargement.
2. Gingival enlargements in pregnancy, puberty are treated with scaling, root planing, and curettage. Enlargements interfering with mastication and esthetics, not subsiding with thorough first phase of therapy should be excised.
3. Drug-induced enlargements: Substitution with alternative drugs should be tried. If patient does not respond, surgical technique should be employed.
4. Chemical plaque control in combination with mechanical debridement appears to be most effective and is the preferred method of periodontal therapy in leukemic patients.

Small area of enlargement (less than 6 teeth), no bone loss/ horizontal bone loss, abundance of keratinized tissue-gingivectomy.

Large area of enlargement, presence of osseous defects, limited keratinized tissue periodontal flap surgery.

Author's Note

a. *Gingival enlargements are one of the most common encountered clinical conditions.*

b. *An able clinician should at the first visit of a patient reporting with gingival enlargement, perform thorough examination of oral cavity, take medical history and establish a differential diagnosis. It is imperative to recognize the clinical features of each type of enlargements to chart the treatment plan.*

c. *In case of drug-induced enlargements, dentists should perform non-surgical therapy and coordinate with physician to modify/adjust the dosage. In moderate to advanced cases, surgical treatment can be done. Patient should be given oral hygiene instructions.*

d. *Pregnancy and pubertal enlargements should be treated in conservative manner at recall visits.*

e. *Periodontal abscesses are usually mistaken for periapical abscess by practitioners. Deep periodontal pocket and radiographic evidence of absence of caries is a diagnostic criterion for periodontal abscess.*

f. *Exostosis and Tori should not be a concern unless they impose functional/esthetic problems.*

Internal Bevel Gingivectomy for Amlodipine-induced Gingival Overgrowth (Fig. 3.6a to j)

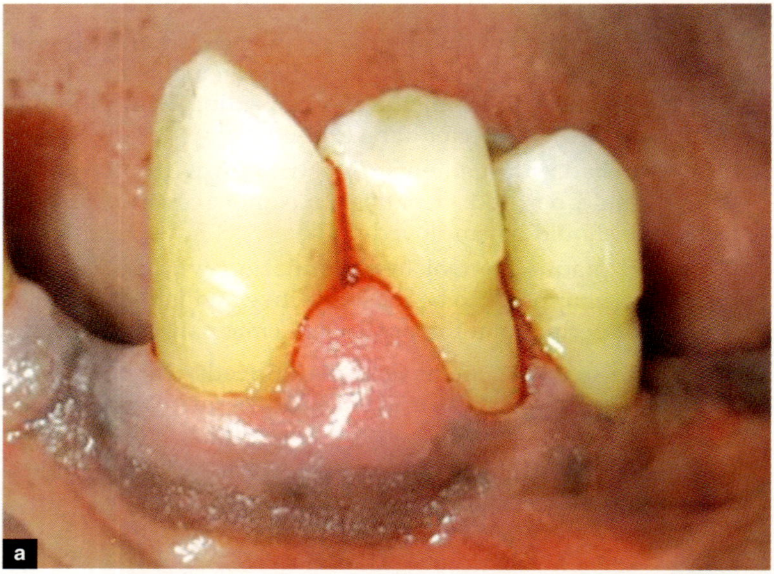

a

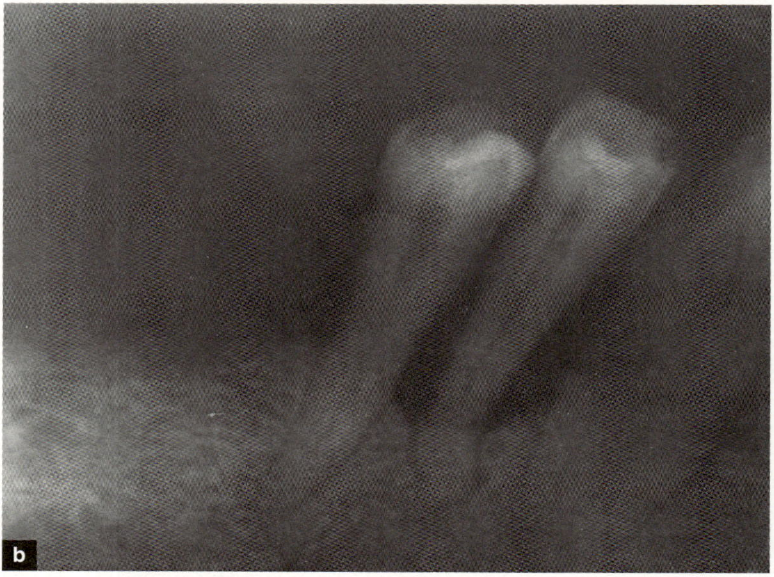

b

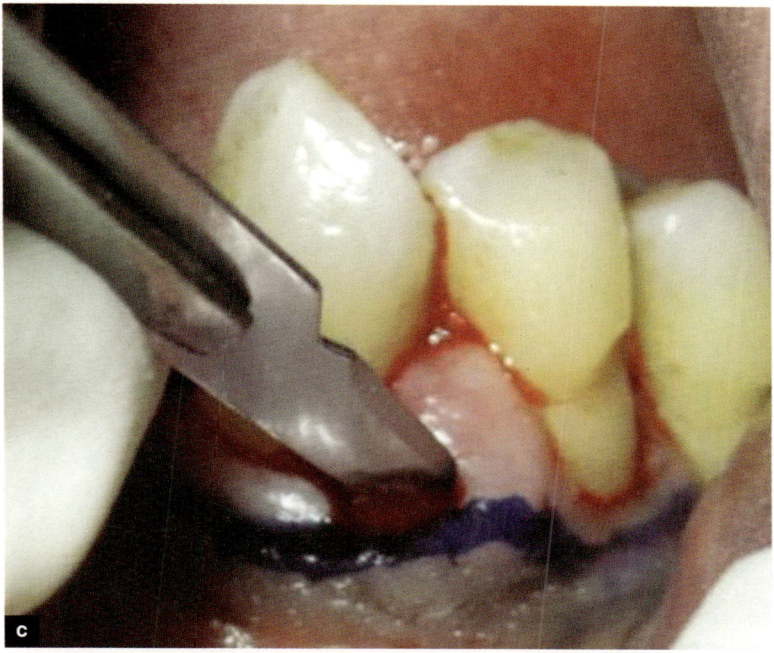

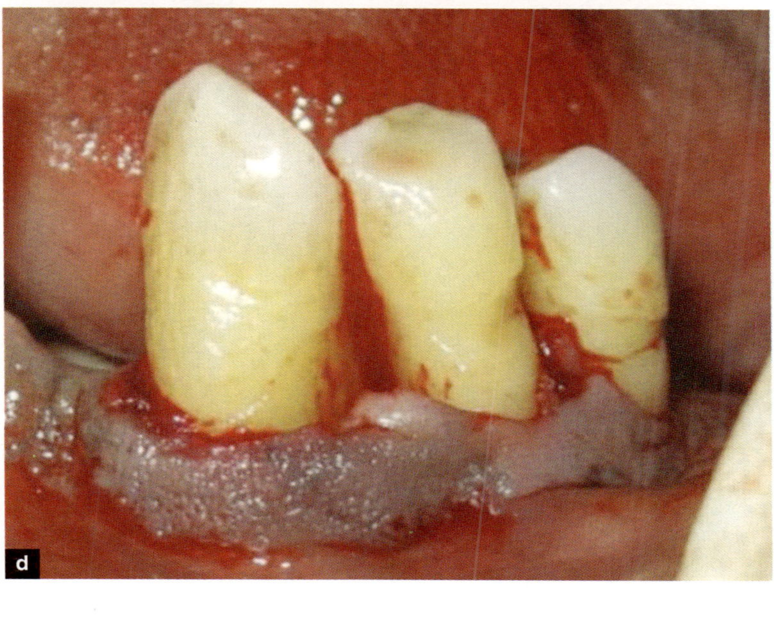

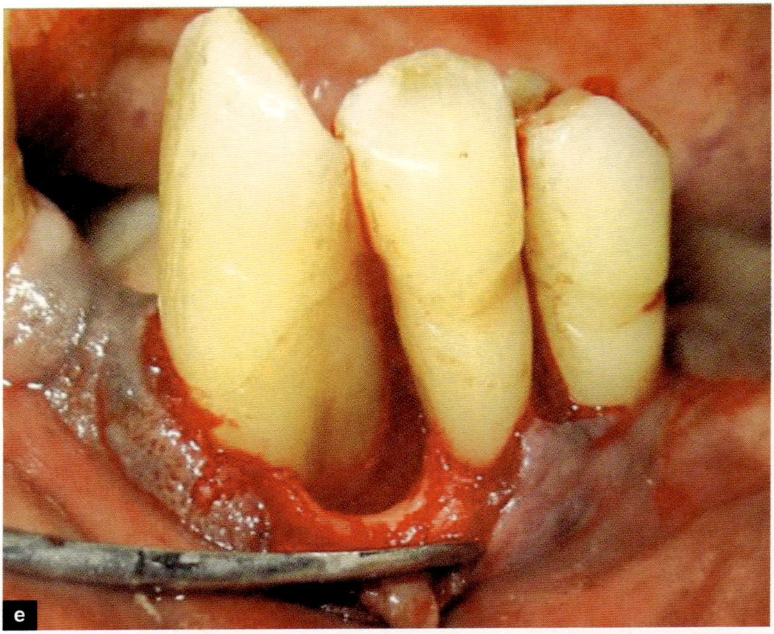

e

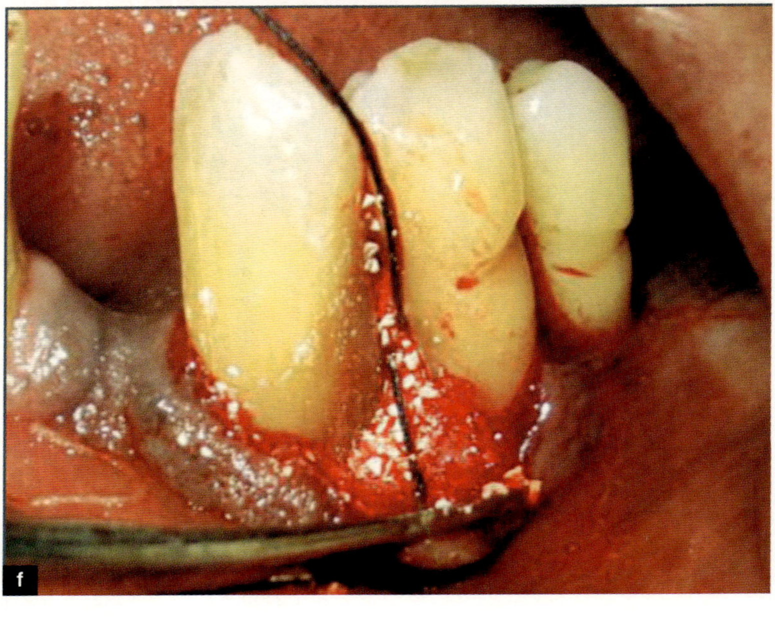

f

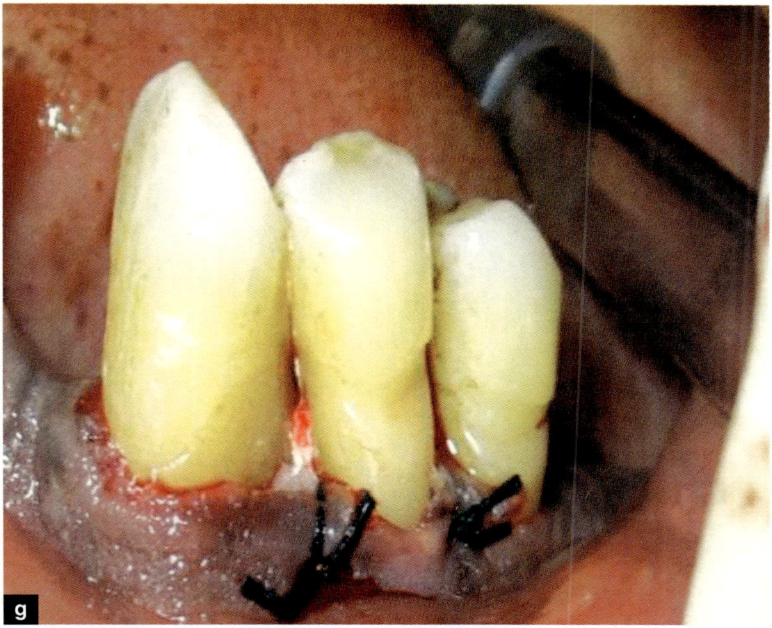

g

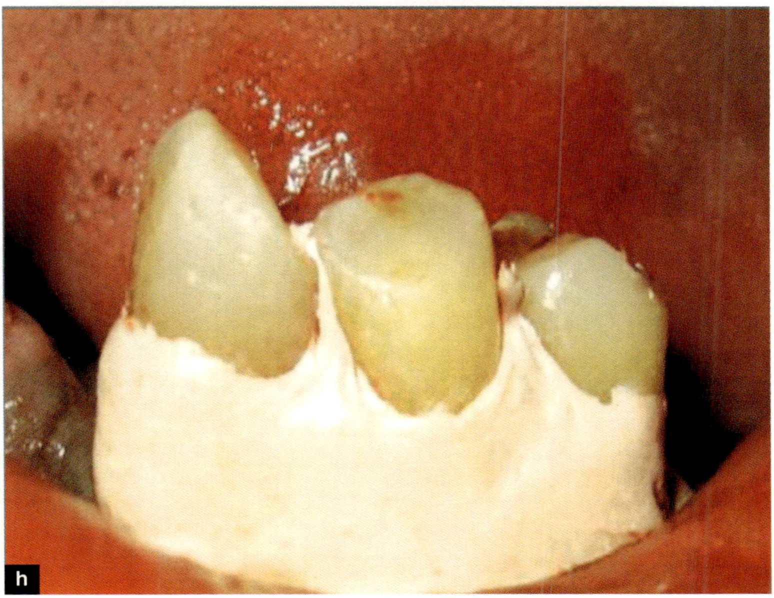

h

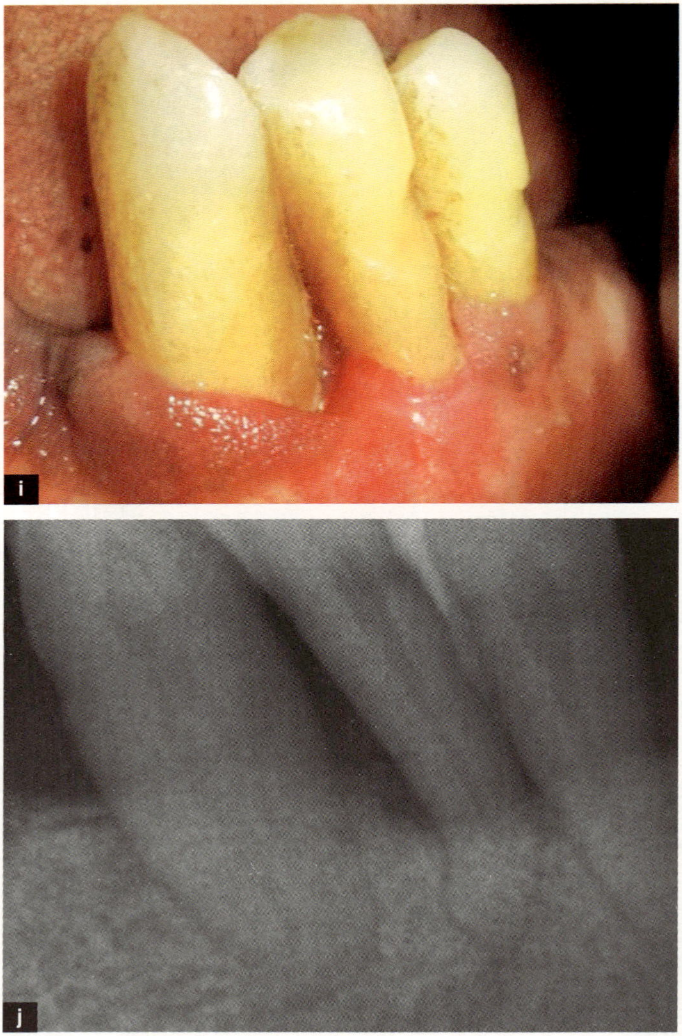

Fig. 3.6a to j: (a) Gingival enlargement 33,34; (b) IOPA showing intrabony defect; (c) Interna bevel incision to preserve the tissue. Incisions made with #15 blade; (d) Excision of gingival overgrowth done; (e) Open flap debridement of two-walled defect; (f) Placement of calcium hydroxyapetite; (g) Placement of sutures; (h) Coe pack placed; (i) Postoperative view after 3 months. (j) Bone fill can be seen in radiograph

4

Acute Gingival Infections

Necrotizing gingivitis (NG), necrotizing periodontitis (NP), and necrotizing stomatitis (NS) are the most severe inflammatory periodontal disorders.

> **Note:** *Usually run an acute course and, therefore, the term acute is often included in the diagnosis.*

NG should be limited to lesions only involving gingival tissue with no loss of periodontal attachment, whereas NP is the terminology used when the lesions involve the periodontal tissues including gingiva, periodontal ligament, and alveolar bone.

ANUG

Acute necrotizing ulcerative gingivitis (ANUG) is also called Vincent's gingivitis or Vincent's gingivostomatitis, necrotizing gingivostomatitis, and trench mouth.

> **Note:** *Cancrum oris, also denoted Noma, is a destructive and necrotizing, frequently fatal stomatitis in which the same mixed fusospirochetal flora as that of ANUG.*

Signs of ANUG

a. Diagnostic feature: Ulcerated and necrotic papillae and gingival margins resulting in a characteristic punched-out appearance.
a. It occurs at all ages, highest incidence between ages 20 and 30 years.
b. The initial signs of lesions are often seen interproximally in the mandibular anterior region, but they may occur in any interproximal space.

> **Note:** *Ulcers are covered by "pseudomembrane". The sloughed material has no coherence, and bears little resemblance to a membrane.*

c. Spontaneous gingival hemorrhage/bleeding on slight provocation.
d. The lesions are seldom associated with deep pocket formation.
e. Sequestrum formation (necrotic bone) in immunocompromised patients.
f. Diagnosis of ANUG is based on clinical findings of gingival. pain, ulceration and bleeding.

Note: *Intact junctional epithelium is needed for pocket formation. In ANUG, extensive gingival necrosis happens and hence no pocket formation.*

Clinical Note

Linear erythema: The zone between the marginal necrosis and the relatively unaffected gingiva usually exhibits a well demarcated narrow erythematous zone. This could be attributed to hyperemia, due to dilation of the vessels in the gingival connective tissue in the periphery of the necrotic lesions.

Symptoms

a. Constant gnawing radiating pain,
b. Extremely sensitive to touch lesions,
c. Metallic foul taste. Pronounced *fetor ex ore* is often associated with NPD but is not pathognomonic only of NPD.
d. Excessive amount of pasty saliva.

Classifications

Horning and Cohen, 1995
Pindborg et al, 1966

Classification by Pindborg et al, 1966

1. Erosion at the tip of interdental papilla
2. Lesion extending to marginal gingiva
3. Lesion extending to attached gingiva
4. Exposure of bone

Classification by Horning and Cohen, 1995

Stage 1: Necrosis of the tip of interdental papilla
Stage 2: Necrosis of entire papilla
Stage 3: Necrosis extending to gingival margin

Stage 4: Necrosis extending to attached gingiva
Stage 5: Necrosis extending into labial or buccal mucosa
Stage 6: Necrosis exposing alveolar bone
Stage 7: Necrosis perforating skin of cheek

Etiology

a. ANUG is caused by fusospirochetal complex; the predominant spirochete isolated is *T. microdentium*. Spirochetes are found as deep as 300 microns from the surface.
b. Loesche *et al.* (1982): Constant flora primarily composed of *Treponema* sp., *Selenomonas* sp., *Fusobacterium* sp., and *B. melaninogenicus* sp, *Prevotella intermedia*, and the variable flora consist of a heterogeneous array of bacterial types.
c. Psychosomatic factors are the most important predisposing factor.
d. Schwartzman reaction refers to effects of endotoxins which are more prominent in NPD than in chronic gingivitis and periodontitis **(Lindhe, 3rd ed)**.

Zones Found in ANUG Lesion (Listgarten, 1965)

1. Bacterial zone
2. Neutrophil rich zone
3. Necrotic zone
4. Spirochetal infiltration zone

Clinical Note

NUG is transmissible (maintenance of an infectious agent in successive passages through a susceptible animal host), not contagious (maintenance of infection by natural modes of contact like air, water, food).

Treatment Phases of ANUG

Treatment of acute gingival infections consists of alleviating the acute inflammation by removal of necrotic tissue, and correction of underlying chronic conditions/systemic diseases.

Treatment is completed in three visits:

a. *First visit:* Removal of necrotic pseudomembrane. Removal of superficial calculus with ultrasonic scaling, subgingival scaling and curettage. Antibiotics in patients with systemic complications. Instructions for 3% hydrogen peroxide rinses and 0.12% chlorhexidine rinses twice daily.

b. *Second visit:* Performed after 1–2 days of initial visit. Shrinkage of gingiva is seen, scaling is done to remove the previously covered calculus.

c. *Third visit:* At 5 days after second visit. Scaling and root planing is done. Patient instructed on nutrition and smoking cessation. Hydrogen peroxide rinses are discontinued. Appointments scheduled for treatment of periodontal pockets and eliminate local sources of irritation.

Primary Herpetic Gingivostomatitis

Clinical features: Infection of the oral cavity caused by herpes simplex virus type I.

a. Asymptomatic primary infection
b. Secondary manifestations: Herpes labialis, herpetic stomatitis, herpetic genitalis, ocular herpes and herpetic encephalitis.
c. Characteristic features are vesicles which rupture to form small, painful shallow ulcers. Primary herpetic gingivitis usually may occur without overt vesciculation.
d. Characteristic symptom: Generalized soreness of the oral cavity which interferes with eating, drinking and oral hygiene.

Histology: Tzank cells (epithelial cells which show ballooning degeneration).

Treatment: An antiviral medication alters the course of the disease.

Note: *Difference between herpetic ulcers and aphthous ulcers is that the diffuse involvement of gingiva does not occur in aphthous ulcers. Primary herpetic gingivostomatitis is contagious.*

Pericoronitis (Fig. 4.1)

Inflammation of the gingiva in relation to the crown of an incompletely erupted tooth.

Operculum: Space between crown and overlying gingival flap.

Complications: Pericoronal abscess, oropharyngeal infection, peritonsillar abscess, cellulitis, Ludwig's angina.

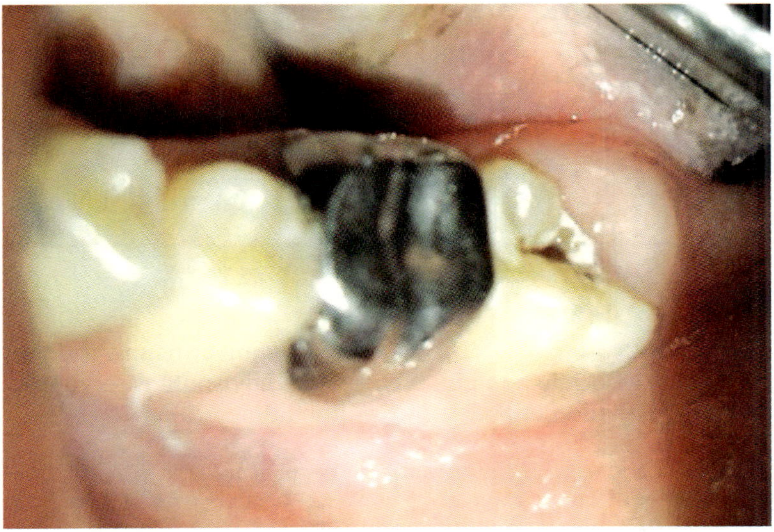

Fig. 4.1: Pericoronitis in relation to incompletely erupted tooth

Note: *When to extract a third molar depends on:*

1. *Inclination of third molar and its relation with second molar*
2. *Amount of bone loss with respect to second molar*
3. *Endodontic involvement of the second molar*

5 Desquamative Gingivitis

Desquamative gingivitis (DG): Defined as an unusual, unique, nonplaque associated gingivitis characterized by intense erythema and desquamation of the surface epithelium.

> ***Note:*** *McCarthy and Shklar for the first time concluded that DG is not a specific entity but is gingival response associated with a variety of conditions (immunopathologic).*

McCarthy and Shklar's classification: Based on etiological considerations, desquamative gingivitis can be the manifestation of:

a. Dermatoses: Lichen planus (Fig. 5.1), mucous membrane pemphigoid, bullous pemphigoid, pemphigus
b. Endocrine imbalance (estrogen deficiency in females menopause/hysterectomy), testosterone deficiency in males previously considered
c. Senile atrophic gingivitis (aging)—not accepted any more
d. Metabolic disturbances (Gingivosis)—not accepted any more
e. Abnormal response to irritation (Toxic—antimetabolites, allergic—barbiturates, antibiotics, etc.)—not accepted
f. Idiopathic
g. Chronic infections: Tuberculosis, chronic candidiasis, histoplasmosis.
h. Drug reactions: Now grouped under lichenoid reactions

Etiology of desquamative gingivitis (at present): Majority of the cases are oral lichen planus (OLP), mucous membrane pemphigoid (MMP) and pemphigus vulgaris (PV) in the same order.

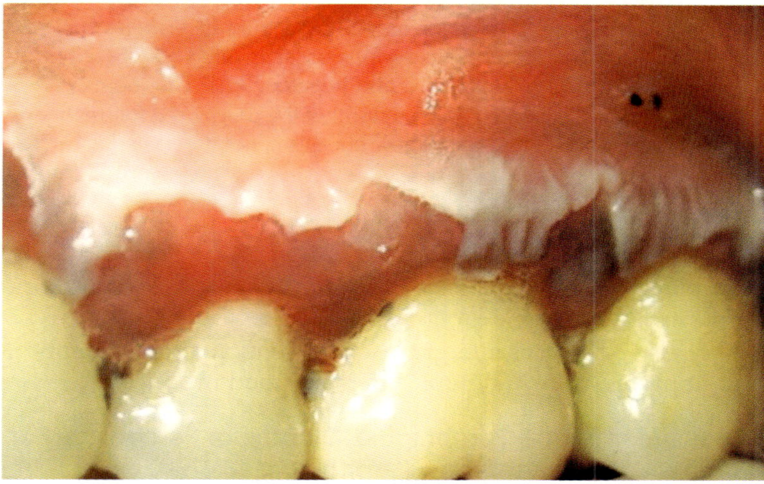

Fig. 5.1: Oral lichen planus

Glickman and Smulow classification: Three forms of desquamative gingivitis: Mild, moderate and severe.

1. Mild form:
   a. Diffuse erythema, some blanching may be seen.
   b. Painless
   c. May complain of intolerance to hot and spicy foods.
2. Moderate form:
   a. Smooth, shiny, soft gingiva, with patchy distribution of bright red and grey areas
   b. Burning sensation
   c. Sensitive to temperature. Inhalation of air may be painful
   d. Massaging the gingiva results in peeling of the epithelium, with bleeding.
3. Severe form:
   a. Wide areas of the oral cavity involved
   b. Very painful.
   c. Surface epithelium appears shredded, blowing of air causes a bubble in gingival epithelium.

Note: *Atypical location and absence of bilateral occurrence are the* differentiating factors from regular OLP.

Grinspan's syndrome: It is characterized by a triad of *diabetes mellitus* (DM), hypertension and oral lichen planus. It is often associated with liver diseases including hepatitis C and hepatocellular carcinoma.

Oral lichen planus is thought to be a result of the drugs used for treatment of hypertension and diabetes mellitus but this is not confirmed.

Oral Mucosa Lichenoid Lesions

These can be attributed to:

1. Systemic drugs such as NSAIDs, β blockers, ACE inhibitors, antimalarial, etc.
2. May also be seen as allergic reactions to monomer, contents of toothpastes, chewing gums and many food products.

Mucous Membrane Pemphigoid/Cicatricial Pemphigoid or Benign Mucous Membrane Pemphigoid (BMMP)

Pathogenesis: Antigen–antibody complex interaction at basement membrane results in complement and leukocyte release of proteolytic enzymes, which cleaves the basement membrane (lamina lucida).

Antigenic determinants: Bullous pemphigoid 1 (BP1) 230 kD protein (most often) and BP2 180 kD protein.

Subtypes: Oral pemphigoid, anti-epiligrin pemphigoid, anti-BP antigen mucosal pemphigoid, ocular pemphigoid and multiple antigens pemphigoid.

Characteristic features: Ocular lesions are the first sign characterized by: Symblepharon (adhesion of eyelid to eyeball), ankyloblepharon (adhesion at the edges of eyelids).

Pemphigus Vulgaris (Others are Pemphigus Foliaceous, Pemphigus Vegetans, Pemphigus Erythematosus)

It is an autoimmune, intraepithelial blistering disease.

Pathogenesis: Autoantibodies against cell surface glycoprotein.

Characteristic features:

a. Tombstone appearance (loss of entire superficial esp.), acantholysis, Nikolsky's sign positive.
b. Oral lesions are the first sign in 60% cases (soft palate commonly, gingival tissues less common)

Note: *Desmoglein 3 correlates with oral disease and desmoglein 1 with cutaneous disease.*

Supportive Measures in the Management of DG

a. Steroids are the mainstay of the treatment.
b. Other alternatives: Photopheresis, plasmapheresis, free gingival graft, laser application.

Note: *Drug eruptions occur due to mercurial compounds, tartar control toothpastes, pyrophosphates, flavoring agents, cinnamon compounds.*

Lesions Mimicking Desquamative Gingivitis

Factitious lesions, candidiasis, graft vs. host disease, Wegener's granulomatosis, Kindler syndrome (cutaneous neonatal bulla, poikiloderma, photosensitivity, acral atrophy).

6 Periodontal Pocket

DEFINITION

A periodontal pocket is a pathologically deepened gingival sulcus (Glickman).

Pseudo or gingival pocket occurs by the coronal movement of the marginal gingiva.

Clinical Features

Symptoms

a. Localized pain or a sensation of pressure in the gingiva after eating, which gradually diminishes.
b. A foul taste in localized areas.
c. A tendency to suck material from the interproximal spaces.
d. Radiating pain deep in the bone.
e. A gnawing feeling or feeling of itching in the gums.
f. The urge to dig a pointed object into the gums with relief from the resultant bleeding.
g. Patient complains that food sticks between the teeth or that the teeth feel loose or a preference to eat on the other side.
h. Sensitivity to heat and cold; toothache in the absence of caries.

Clinical Signs

a. Enlarged, bluish red marginal gingiva with a rolled edge separated from the tooth surface.
b. A bluish red vertical zone extending from the gingival margin to the alveolar mucosa.
c. A break in the faciolingual continuity of the interdental gingiva.
d. Shiny, discolored and puffy gingiva associated with exposed root surfaces.

e. Gingival bleeding, purulent exudates from the gingival margin or its appearance to digital pressure on the lateral aspect of the gingival margin.
f. Mobility, extrusion and migration of teeth.
g. The development of diastema.

Classification of Pockets

1. *Depending upon its morphology* (Fig. 6.1):
   a. Gingival/false/relative pocket/pseudopocket
   b. Periodontal/absolute/true pocket—2 types:
      i. *Suprabony/supracrestal:* Base of pocket is coronal to level of alveolar bone.
      ii. *Infrabony/intrabony/subcrestal/intra-alveolar:* Base of pocket is apical to alveolar bone.
   c. Combined pocket

   Infrabony pockets can further be classified as (Fig. 6.2):
   i. Based on the number of walls (**Goldman and Cohen**, 1958):
      1. One wall defects also called hemiseptum
      2. Two-walled defects
      3. Three-walled defect/intrabony defect
      4. Combined osseous defect
   ii. According to depth and width:
      1. Shallow and narrow 2. Shallow and wide
      3. Deep and narrow 4. Deep and wide

Note: *Spiral pockets are most common in furcation area.*

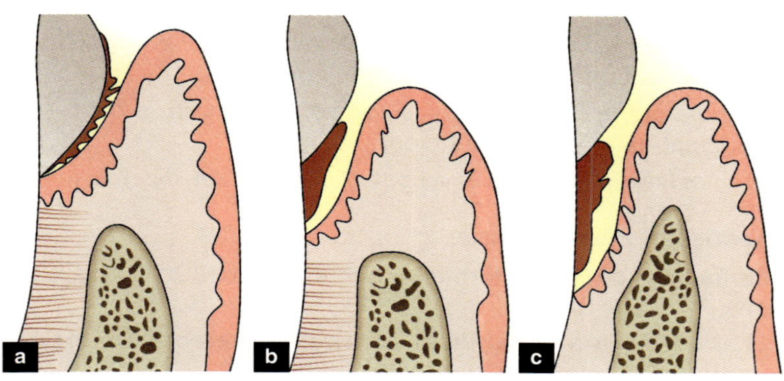

Fig. 6.1a to c: Classification of pocket depending on morphology: (a) Gingival pocket; (b) Suprabony pocket; (c) Infrabony pocket

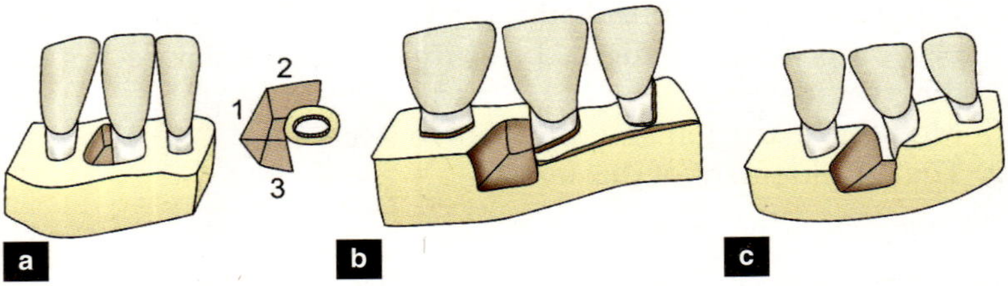

Fig. 6.2a to c: Classification of infrabony defects based on number of walls. (a) One-walled defect; (b) Two-walled defect; (c) Three-walled defect

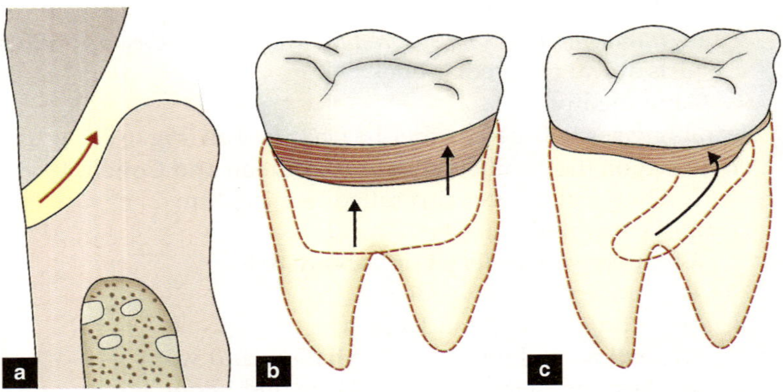

Fig. 6.3a to c: Classification of pocket based on tooth surfaces. (a) Simple pocket; (b) Compound pocket; (c) Complex pocket

2. *Depending upon the number of surfaces involved* (Fig. 6.3): Simple pocket, compound pocket, complex pocket
3. *Depending upon the nature of the soft tissue wall of the pocket:* Edematous pocket, fibrotic pocket
4. *Depending upon the disease activity:* Active pocket, inactive pocket

Theories of Pathogenesis

Ten theories of pocket formation were proposed (Glickman, 8th ed):

1. Destruction of gingival fibers is a prerequisite for the initiation of pocket formation (Fish, 1948).
2. The initial change in pocket formation occurs in the cementum (Gottlieb, 1926).

3. Simulation of the epithelial attachment by inflammation rather than destruction of the gingival fibers is the prerequisite for the initiation of the periodontal pocket (Goldman, 1944).
4. Pathologic destruction of the epithelial attachment due to infection or trauma is the initial histologic change in pocket formation (Skillen, 1930).
5. The periodontal pocket is initiated by invasion of bacteria at the base of the sulcus or the absorption of bacterial toxins at the epithelial lining of the sulcus (Box, 1941).
6. Pocket formation is initiated in a defect in the sulcus wall (Becks, 1929).
7. Proliferation of the epithelium of the lateral wall, rather than the epithelium at the base of the sulcus, is the initial change in the formation of the periodontal pocket (Wilkinson, 1935).
8. Two-stage pocket formation (James and Counsell, 1927).
9. Inflammation is the initial change in the formation of the periodontal pocket (Nukolls and Dienstein).
10. Pathologic epithelial proliferation occurs secondary to non-inflammatory degenerative changes in the periodontal membrane (Aisenberg and Aisenberg).

Clinical Note

The rationale for pocket reduction is based on the need to eliminate areas of plaque accumulation.

Correlation of Clinical and Histopathological Features of a Periodontal Pocket

1. Varying degrees of bluish red discoloration, flaccidity, smooth, shiny surface and pitting on pressure: Discoloration is due to circulatory stasis, flaccidity due to destruction of the gingival fibers, smooth shiny owing to atrophy of epithelium, pitting on pressure due to edema and degeneration.
2. The gingival wall may be pink and firm: Fibrotic changes predominate over exudation and degeneration, particularly in relation to the outer surface of the pocket wall.

Note: *Despite external appearance, internal wall is often ulcerated and presents signs of degeneration. That is the reason bleeding is elicited while probing and not touching the gingival surface of pocket.*

3. Bleeding is elicited by gentle probing the soft tissue wall of the pocket: Increased vascularity, thinning and degeneration of the epithelium and proximity of engorged vessels to the inner surface.
4. When explored with a probe the inner aspect of the pocket is generally painful: Ulceration of the inner aspect of pocket wall.
5. Pus may be expressed by digital pressure: Occurs in pockets with suppurative inflammation of the inner wall.

Note: *When volume of PMNs reaches 60% or more in the junction epithelium, tissue loses cohesiveness and detaches from tooth surface resulting in apical shift, deepening of the gingival sulcus.*

Pocket formation does not occur in ANUG. This happens because necrosis of junctional epithelium (e.g. in ANUG) impairs rather than accelerate pocket formation.

Microtopography of the Gingival Wall of the Pocket

(Saglie, Carranza, Newman et al, 1982).

1. Areas of relative quiescence
2. Areas of bacterial accumulation
3. Areas of emergence of leukocytes
4. Areas of leukocytes bacterial interaction
5. Areas of intense epithelial desquamation
6. Areas of ulceration
7. Areas of hemorrhage

Note: *The most severe degenerative changes in the periodontal pocket occur along the lateral wall.*

The coronoapical length of junctional epithelium at the base of pocket reduces to 50–100 micrometers in length.

Zones in the Bottom of the Periodontal Pocket

1. Cementum covered by calculus where all the changes described earlier takes place.
2. Attached plaque which covers calculus (100–500 μ).
3. The zone of unattached plaque.
4. The zone where the junctional epithelium is attached to the tooth. This zone, which is normally more than 500 μ is usually reduced to less than 100 μ in periodontal pocket.
5. Apical to the junctional epithelium there may be a zone of semi-destroyed connective tissue fibres.

Areas 3, 4, and 5 compose the so-called plaque-free zone and refer only to attached plaque.

Different Patterns of Bone Loss

Garant and Cho (1979) were the first to point out that bone resorption occurs within a finite radius of action.

Radius of action: Waerhaug measured the distance between the attached plaque to bone and found it to be never less than 0.5 mm and never more than 2.7 mm. Bone resorbing activity induced by the bacteria is exerted within these distances.

Clinical Note

Why different kinds of bone loss in different areas?

In areas of thin alveolar housing on the facial and lingual aspects of teeth: Apical extension of plaque would cause destruction of the entire thickness of the alveolar process rather than cause pockets.

In areas of bone thickness greater than 2 mm: Angular craters can form in bone in the interdental and inter-radicular areas and cause uneven areas of vertical and horizontal bone loss.

Clinical Note

Severity of bone loss cannot always be correlated with pocket depth (Fig. 6.4).

In cases of gingival recession, extensive attachment and bone loss may be associated with shallow pockets and vice versa.

Pocket depth is the distance between base of the pocket and crest of gingival margin. Loss of attachment (LOA) is the distance between the cementoenamel junction and base of sulcus.

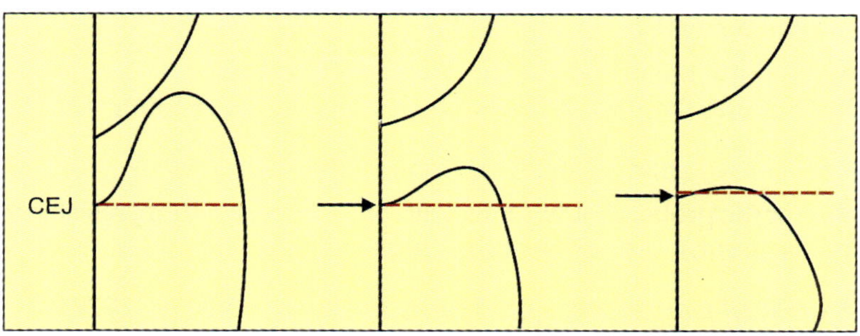

Fig. 6.4: Different pocket depths with same amount of attachment loss (CEJ is a constant factor, the base of the pocket varies)

Determination of Pocket Depth

a. Probing depth measurement.
b. Clinical detection of attachment loss

Diagnosis of pockets: The only accurate method of detecting and evaluating periodontal pockets is careful exploration with a pocket probe.

Hirschfield in 1953 used gutta-percha points or calibrated silver points with the X-ray to assist in determining the level of the attachment of periodontal pockets and their relationship to the bone.

Clinical Note

Pockets are not detected or measured by radiographic examination. The periodontal pocket is a soft tissue change. Radiographs indicate bone loss where pockets may be suspected.

Pocket Probing

There are two different pocket depths:

1. *Biologic or histologic pocket depth:* Distance between the gingival margin and the bottom of the pocket, i.e. the coronal end of the junctional epithelium. This can be measured only in carefully prepared histologic sections. Ranges from 0 to 6 mm (average 1.8 mm).
2. *Clinical or probing pocket depth:* Distance to which an ad-hoc instrument or probe penetrates into the pocket depth. Average 2–3 mm.

Method of Probing (Fig. 6.5)

a. Walking the probe: To check for probing depth
b. Running the probe: To check for bleeding on probing

Factors Affecting Depth of Penetration of a Probe

Size of the probe, probing force, direction of penetration, resistance of the tissues, convexity of the crown

Depth of penetration of a probe (Armitage et al, 1977)

a. In healthy specimens, the probe penetrates the epithelium to about two-thirds of its length.

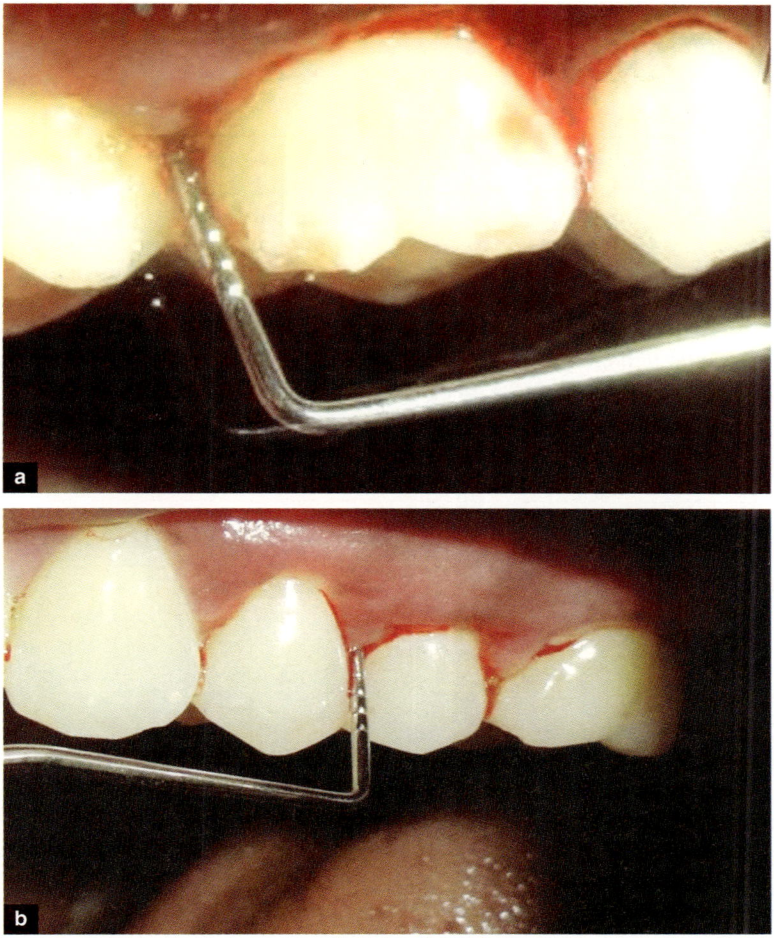

Fig. 6.5a and b: The periodontal probe should be held parallel to long axis of tooth

b. In gingivitis specimens, it stopped 0.1 mm short of its apical end.
c. In periodontitis specimens, the probe tip consistently went past the most apical cells of the junctional epithelium.
d. The depth of penetration of a probe in the connective tissue apical to the junctional epithelium in a periodontal pocket is about 0.3 mm.

The forces of 0.75N have been found to be well tolerated and accurate for probing.

Author's Note

a. *At an undergraduate level, differentiating between a deep normal sulcus and a shallow periodontal pocket is a difficult and confusing task. In such a case, a decision should be made by looking at the pathologic features in gingiva, the force used to probe and soft tissue resistance felt while probing. These cumulative features will also help in differentiating gingivitis from periodontitis.*
b. *Minimal force should be applied while probing (equivalent to pricking the tip of finger to draw blood)*
c. *Tactile perception in a dental physician is most important asset to determine the type of periodontal pocket clinically.*
d. *Shallow pockets subside after a good non-clinical therapy. Treatments of deep pockets with bone defects are discussed in next chapter.*

7

Periodontal Flap and Techniques for Pocket Therapy

Periodontal flap is defined as 'the section of gingiva and/or mucosa surgically elevated from the underlying tissues to provide visibility and access to the bone and root surfaces'.

Rationale of Flap Surgery

a. To enable visual instrumentation of root surfaces
b. Eliminate or reduce pocket depth by resection of pocket wall
c. Gain access for osseous resective surgery, if necessary
d. Expose the area to perform regenerative methods

Indications of Flap Surgery

Primarily in cases of periodontitis with active pockets >5 mm, which does not respond to initial non-surgical therapy.

Historical Background

Neumann (1911)	1st introduced mucoperiosteal flap—Neumann flap
Cieszynski (1911)	Reverse bevel incision
Leonard Widman (1918)	Modified Neumann flap
Kirkland (1931)	Modified flap procedure
Nabers (1954)	Introduced 'repositioning of attached gingiva'
Ariaudo and Tyrell (1962)	Modified Nabers procedure
Friedman (1962)	Apically positioned flap
Morris (1965)	Unrepositioned mucoperiosteal flap
Ramfjord and Nissle (1974)	Modified Widman flap

Classification of Flaps

1. *Based on bone exposure after flap reflection (Fig. 7.1):* Full thickness flap (mucoperiosteal flap) and partial thickness flap (split thickness/mucosal)
2. *Based on flap placement after surgery:*
   a. Undisplaced (non-displaced/unrepositioned): Modified Widman flap, undisplaced flap

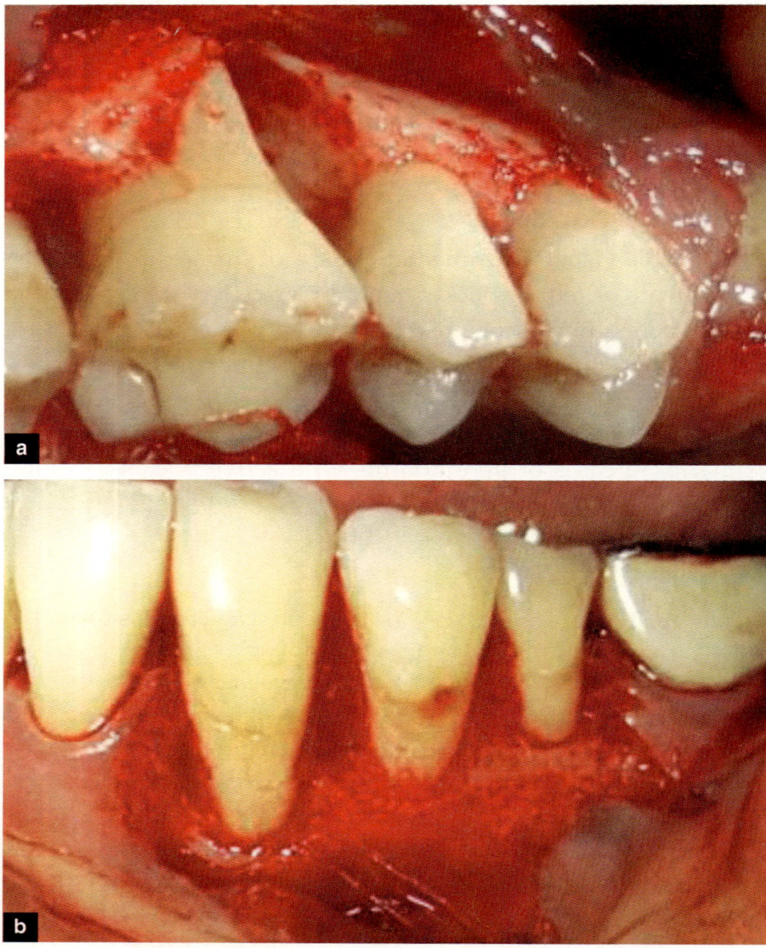

Fig. 7.1a and b: (a) Full thickness flap; (b) Partial thickness flap

Clinical Note

To displace flap, attached gingiva is totally separated from underlying bone, enabling the mobility of unattached gingiva.

Palatal flaps cannot be displaced because of the absence of unattached gingiva.

   b. Displaced (repositioned): Coronally positioned, laterally positioned, apically positioned flap
   c. Undisplaced flap (excisional procedure) removes the pocket wall, reduces/eliminates the pocket.
   d. Apically displaced flap apically positions soft tissue wall of pocket, eliminates the pocket, and increases the width of attached gingiva (transforms unattached keratinized pocket wall into attached tissue).

3. *Based on the management of papilla:*
   a. Conventional flaps: Modified Widman flap, undisplaced flap, apically displaced flap, flap for reconstructive procedures.
      Technique: Papilla is split at center beneath contact point and included in both buccal and palatal/lingual flaps.
   b. Papilla preservation flap: Papilla is included in one of the flaps by semicircular incision.

Clinical Note

Modified Widman flap is not intended to eliminate or reduce pocket depth. It removes the pocket lining and reduction in pocket depth occurs due to tissue shrinkage.

Note: *Difference between original and modified Widman flap.*
Technique in original Widman flap included both apical displacement of the flaps and osseous recontouring (elimination of bony defects) to obtain proper pocket elimination. In modified Widman flap, the flaps are approximated to cover the entire tissue, thus causing less exposure of root surfaces.

Incisions

1. **Horizontal incisions (Fig. 7.2a and b):** This is directed along the margin of the gingiva in mesial/distal direction. Two types:
   a. *Internal bevel incision/reverse bevel incision:* It is the first incision and basic to periodontal surgeries. Made with #15,

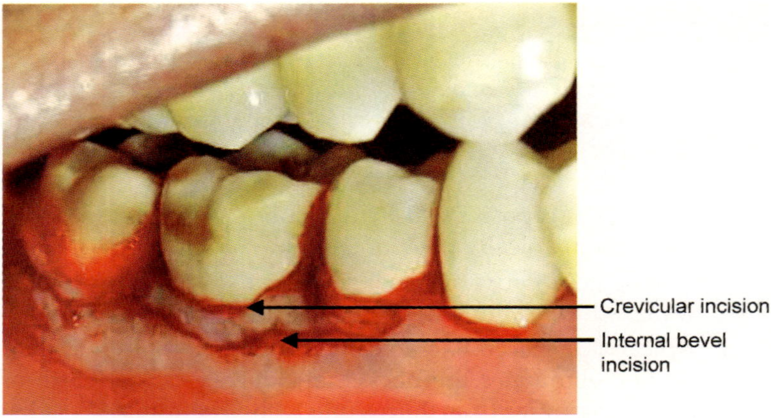

Fig. 7.2a: Position of crevicular and internal bevel incisions

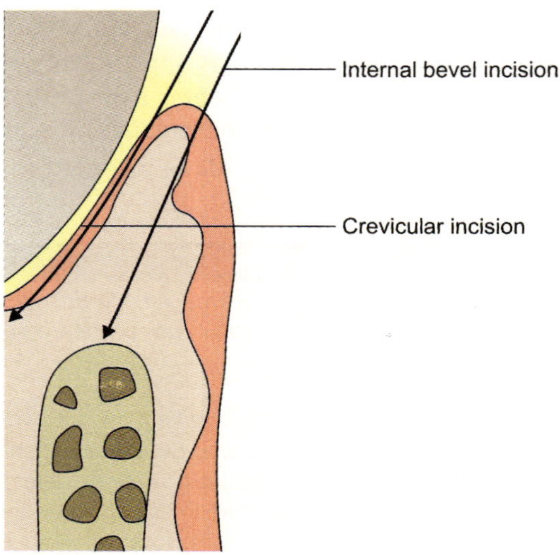

Fig. 7.2b: Diagram depicting the horizontal incision markings

#15 C. Incision is made at the distance from gingival margin till bone crest. Aims at: (i) Removing the pocket lining; (ii) Conserves the uninvolved outer surface of the gingiva; (iii) Produces sharp flap margin for adaptation to bone–tooth junction.

b. *Crevicular incision:* It is the second incision. Made with #12D. Incision starts from the base of pocket to the crest of the bone.
c. *Interdental incision:* Also called third incision. Made with orban knife.

2. **Vertical incision (Fig. 7.3a and b):** Vertical/oblique releasing incisions are made at ends of horizontal incisions, if flaps are to be displaced.

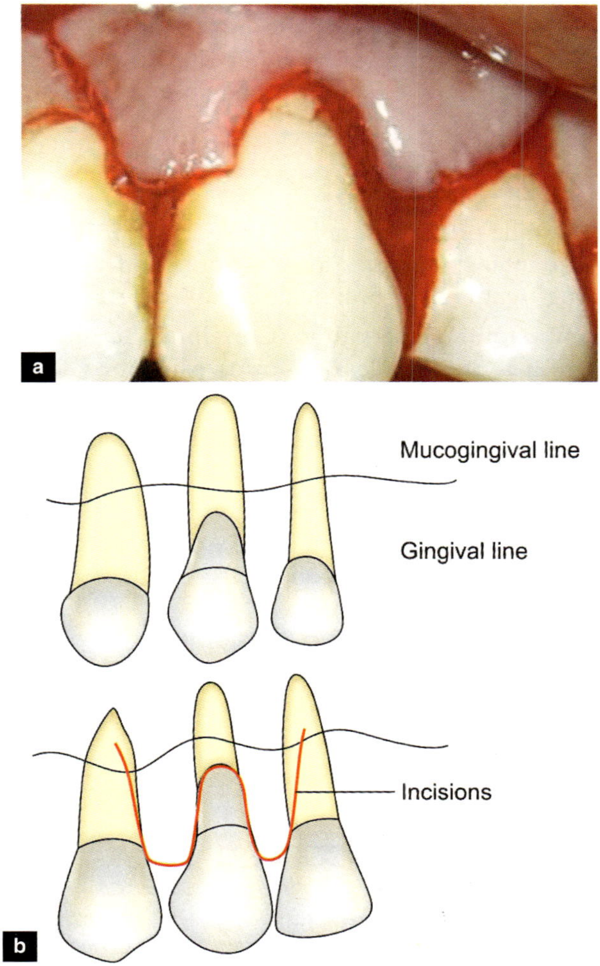

Fig. 7.3a and b: Vertical incisions to displace the flap

Types of Incisions in Various Flap Surgeries

a. *Modified Widman flap:* Incision is made close to the gingival margin (1–2 mm) for the removal of pocket lining.

b. *Apically displaced flap:* Incision is made as close to the tooth as possible (0.5–1 mm). Removal of pocket lining and preservation of the keratinized gingiva.

c. *Undisplaced flap:* Incision initiated at or near a point coronal to the where the bottom of the pocket is projected on the outer surface of gingiva. Pocket depth and location of mucogingival junction determined to evaluate amount of attached gingiva.

Other Types of Flap Designs

a. Simple papilla preservation flap (Takei et al, 1985): To preserve the interdental soft tissues for maximum soft tissue coverage involving treatment of proximal osseous defects.

b. Modified papilla preservation (Cortellini et al, 1995) used in wide interdental spaces (>2 mm) especially in anterior dentition.

c. Palatal flaps: Oschenbein and Bohannan (1963, 1964) described a palatal approach for osseous surgery.

d. Distal wedge procedure (Robinson, 1966): Indicated when only limited amount of keratinized gingiva is present and in treatment of distal angular bony defects.

Long-Term Studies Comparing Surgical and Non-surgical Therapies

1. Michigan studies (Ramfjord et al., 1968)
2. Michigan studies (Knowles et al.,1979)
3. Gothenburg studies (Lindhe et al., 1982)

Clinical Note

In a full thickness flap, the loss of bone is about 1 mm.

Interdental areas have cancellous bone, and repair results in total restitution without any loss of bone, whereas in radicular bone if bone is thin, there is loss of marginal bone.

4. Minnesota study (Philstrom et al., 1985)
5. Aarhus study (Isidor and Korning, 1986)
6. Washington study (Olsen et al., 1985)
7. Tucson studies (Becker et al., 1988)
8. Nebraska studies (Kaldahl et al., 1988)

Healing after Flap Surgery

1. Immediately after flap surgery, the area between the flap and bone surface is occupied by blood clot which consists of fibrin reticulum with leukocytes, erythrocytes, debris and capillaries at the edges of wound.
2. A week later, blood clot is replaced by granulation tissue.
3. Two weeks after surgery, immature collagen fibres establish weak connection. Clinically, healing appears to be complete.
4. A fully epithelialized gingival crevice with functional arrangement of fibres is complete 1 month after surgery.

Author's Note

a. *Objectives of the type of procedure should determine incisions and final position of the flap.*

b. *Clean incisions, close adaptation of the flap to the underlying bone. Preservation of good blood supply are vital for a successful result.*

c. *In osseous surgeries, flaps should be positioned apically to minimize postoperative pocket depth. Flaps should be reflected to expose at least 3 mm of crestal bone.*

d. *Inadvertent surgeries should not be done, else loss of bone occurs. Bone loss is greater, if bone is thin.*

e. *Complete soft tissue coverage of the alveolar bone should be achieved, not only at buccal/lingual sites but also in proximal sites.*

f. *Care should be taken during surgery to avoid unnecessary tearing of the flaps and to keep the bone moistened with intermittent irrigation to minimize postoperative pain. Pre-emptive analgesia can be done with mild analgesics in apprehensive patients prior to surgery.*

f. *Patient should be instructed for maintenance of optimal postoperative oral hygiene.*

Modified Widman Flap (Fig. 7.4a to h)

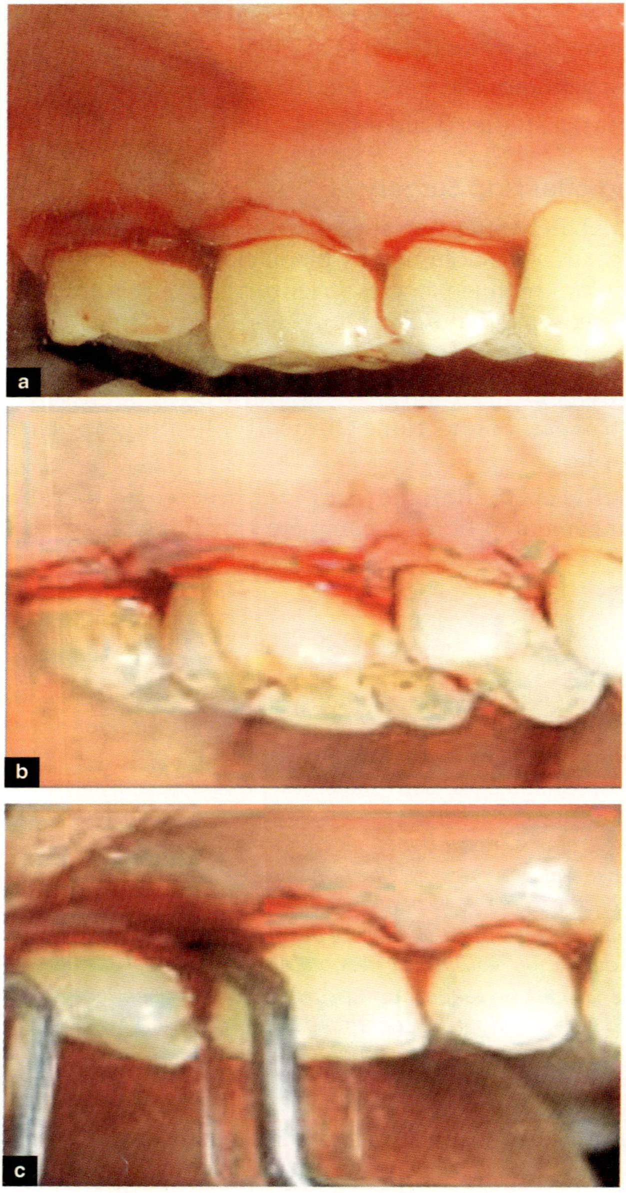

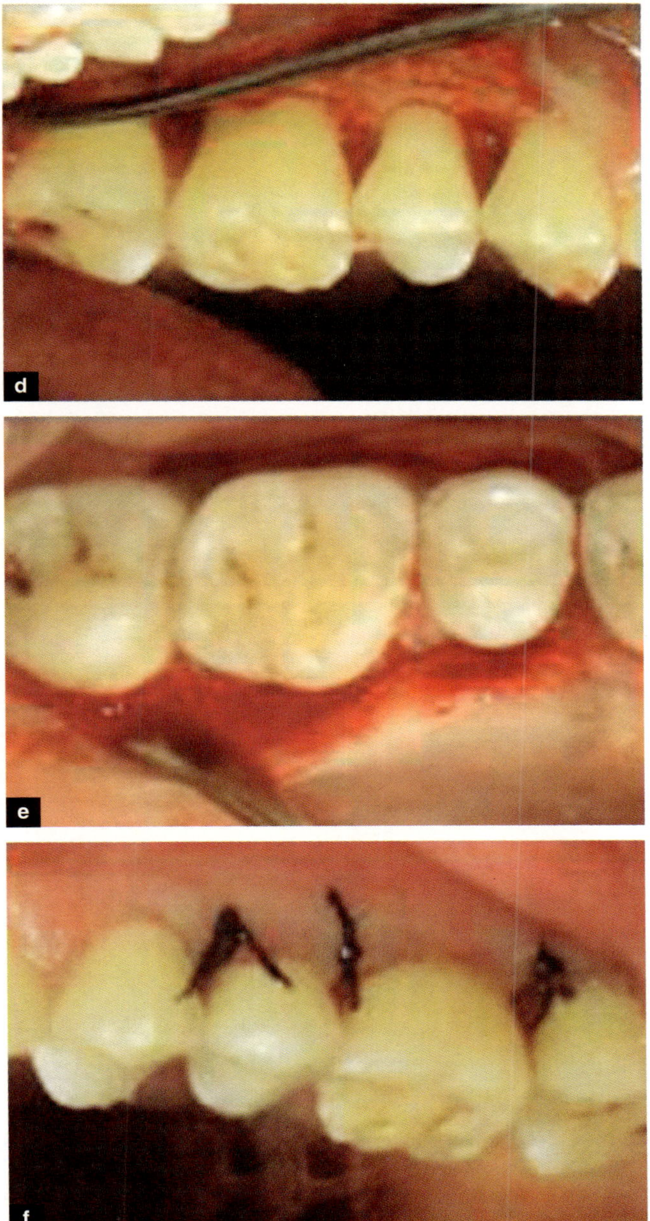

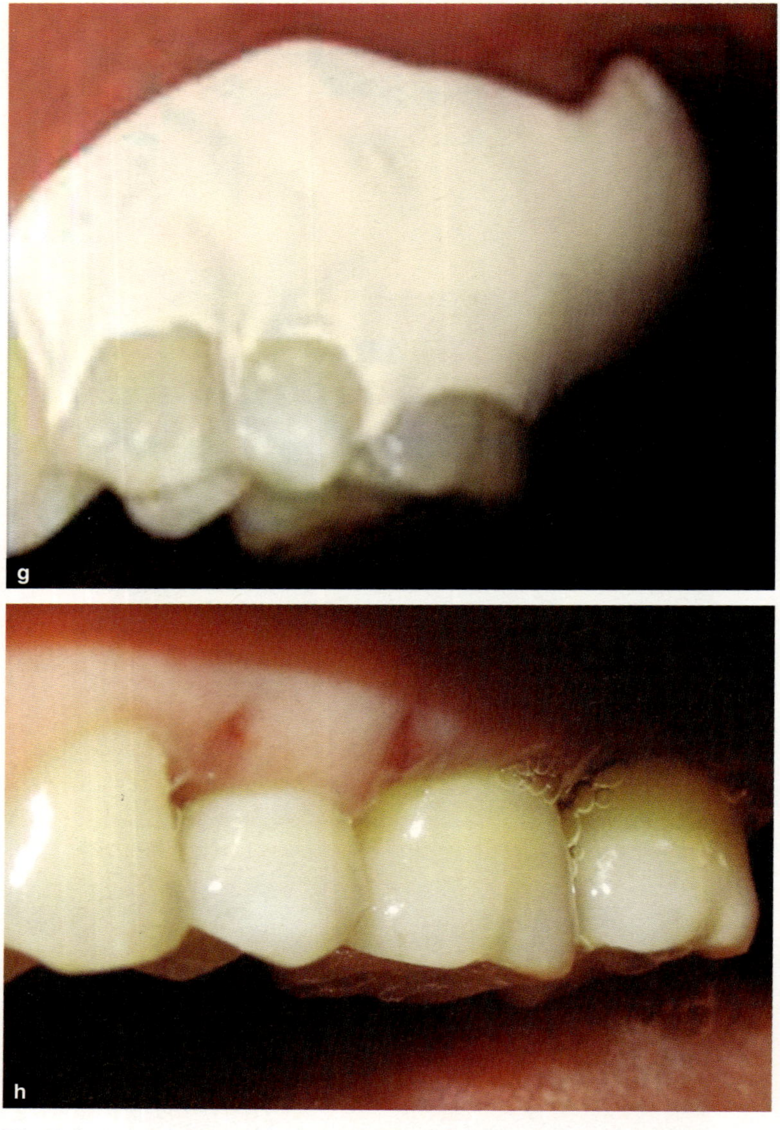

Fig. 7.4a to h: (a) Facial internal bevel incisions; (b) Palatal incisions; (c) Removal of tissue; (d) and (e) Elevation of the flap and; debridement done; (f) Single interrupted suturing done; (g) Periodontal coe-pack placed; (h) Postoperative result

Kirkland Flap (Fig. 7.5a to f)

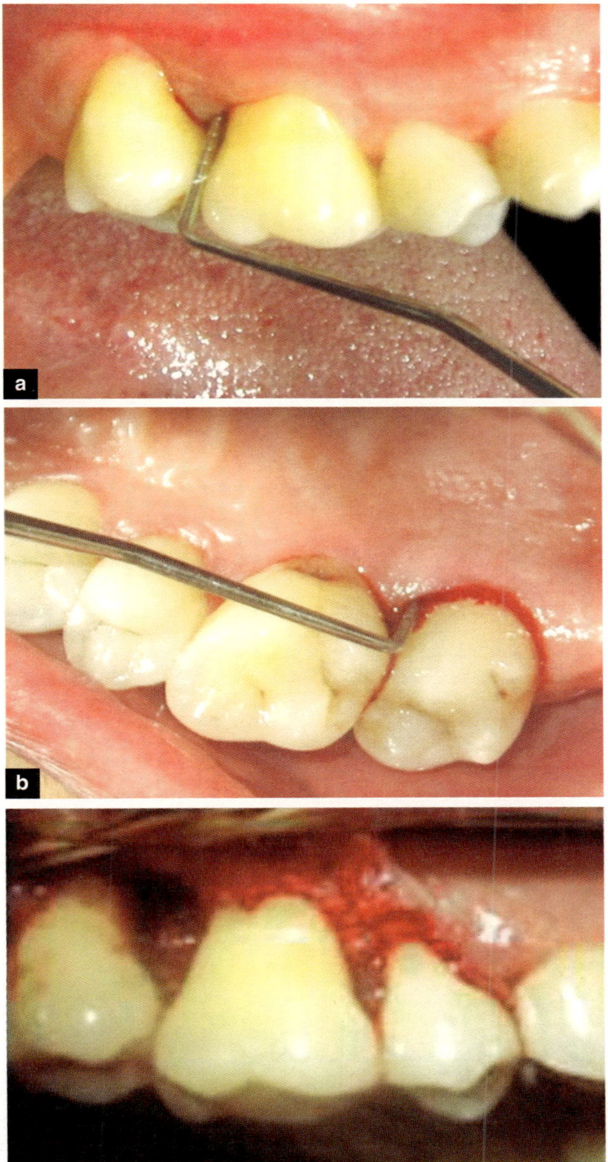

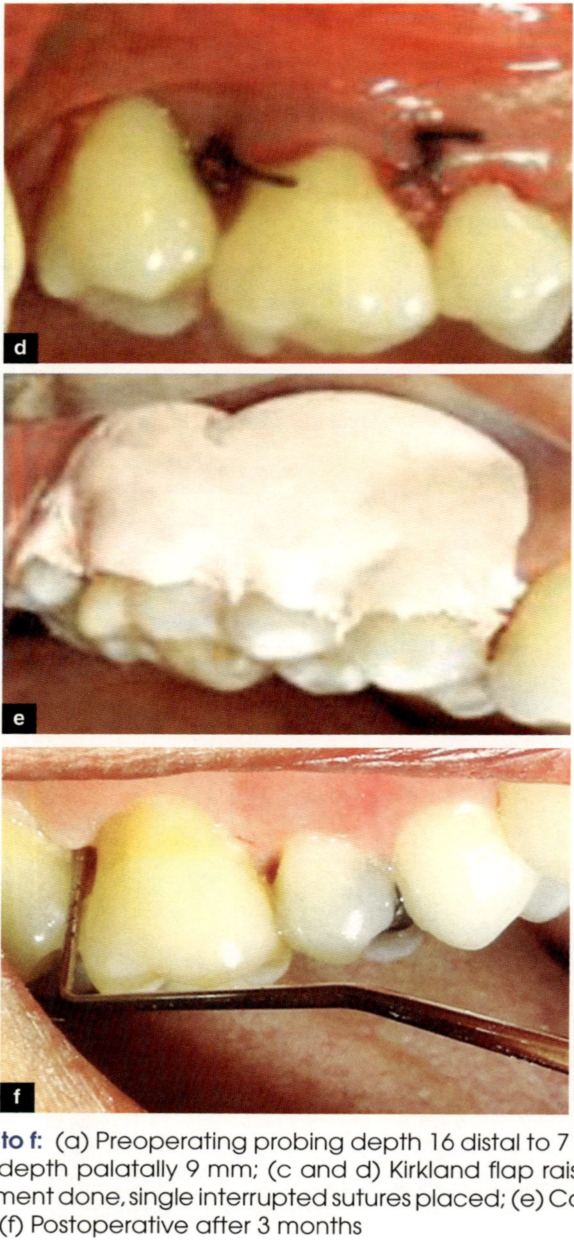

Fig. 7.5a to f: (a) Preoperating probing depth 16 distal to 7 mm; (b) Probing depth palatally 9 mm; (c and d) Kirkland flap raised and debridement done, single interrupted sutures placed; (e) Coe-pack placed; (f) Postoperative after 3 months

8

Resective Osseous Surgery

OSSEOUS SURGERY

Procedure by which changes in alveolar bone can be accomplished to get rid of deformities induced by periodontal disease or other related factors such as exostosis or tooth supraeruption (Carranza, 9th ed).

Classified as

1. **Based on morphologic description:** Additive or subtractive osseous surgery
   a. *Additive osseous surgery:* Procedures directed at restoring alveolar bone to its original level.
   b. *Subtractive osseous surgery:* Restoring the form of pre-existing alveolar bone to the level present at the time of surgery or slightly more apical to the level.
2. **Based on therapeutic result:** Definitive or compromised
   a. *Definitive osseous reshaping:* Further osseous reshaping would not improve the overall result.
   b. *Compromised osseous reshaping:* Bone pattern that cannot be improved without significant osseous removal that would be detrimental to the overall result.
3. **Based on type of surgical technique:** Osteoplasty or ostectomy
   a. *Osteoplasty:* Reshaping the bone without removing tooth supporting bone.
   b. *Ostectomy:* Removal of tooth supporting bone.

Classification of Osseous Defects

A. Glickman (1964)

1. Osseous crater
2. Intrabony defects

3. Bulbous bony contours
4. Hemisepta
5. Inconsistent margins
6. Ledges

B. Karn et al (1984) Topographic Classification

1. Osseous craters
2. Trench
3. Moat
4. Ramp
5. Plane
6. Cratered ramp
7. Ramp into a crater or trench
8. Bulbous bony contours
9. Ledges
10. Reversed architecture
11. Horizontal bone loss
12. Vertical/angular defects

C. Classification of Vertical/Angular Defects

I. Based on number of walls involved:

3-wall defect, 2-wall defect, 1-wall defect/hemisepta, combination: 4-wall defect/moat, trench

II. Depending on the depth and width of the defect

Deep—wide/narrow
Shallow—wide/narrow

Nomenclature of Deformities in Alveolar Bone (Fig. 8.1)

1. *Craters:* A concavity (saucer-shaped) in the interdental bone confined within facial and lingual walls.
2. *Trench:* When crater-like bone loss affects two or three confluent surfaces of the same tooth.
3. *Moat:* When crater-like bone loss involves all four surfaces of tooth it is described as a moat.
4. *Ramp:* The term ramp describes deformity that results when both alveolar bone and its supporting bone are lost to the same

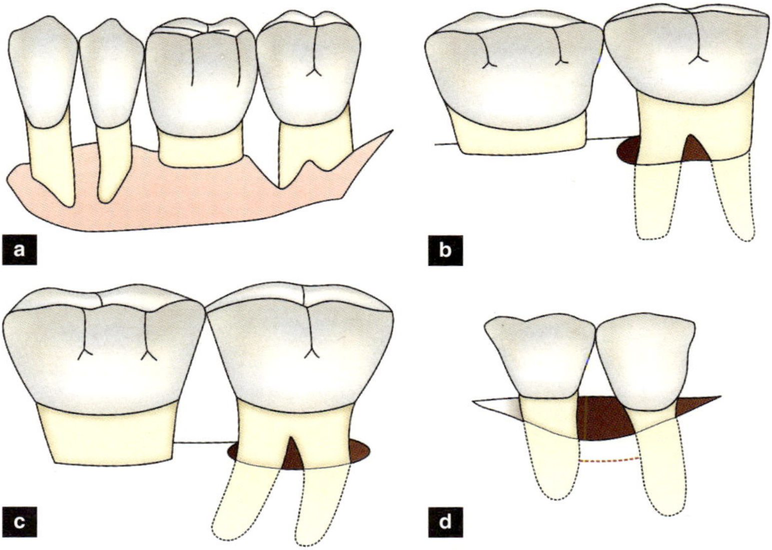

Fig. 8.1a to d: Types of osseous defects; (a) Ramp; (b) Trench; (c) Moat; (d) Cratered ramp

degree in such a manner that the margins of the deformity are at different levels.

5. *Plane:* This term is applied when both alveolar bone and supporting bone are lost to the same degree such that the margins of the deformity are at the same level. It can be considered horizontal bone loss about one tooth or portion of a tooth.
6. *Cratered ramp:* A crater with a portion of its facial and/or lingual wall missing.
7. *Ledges:* Ledges are plateau-like bone margins caused by resorption of thickened bony plates.
8. *Bulbous bony contours:* Bony enlargements caused by exostoses, adaptation to function or buttressing bone formation.

Clinical Note (Fig. 8.2)

Fenestrations: *Isolated areas where root is denuded of bone and covered only by periosteum and overlying gingiva with the marginal bone intact.*

***Dehiscence**: When the denuded areas extend through the marginal bone. More common on anterior teeth and facial bone.*

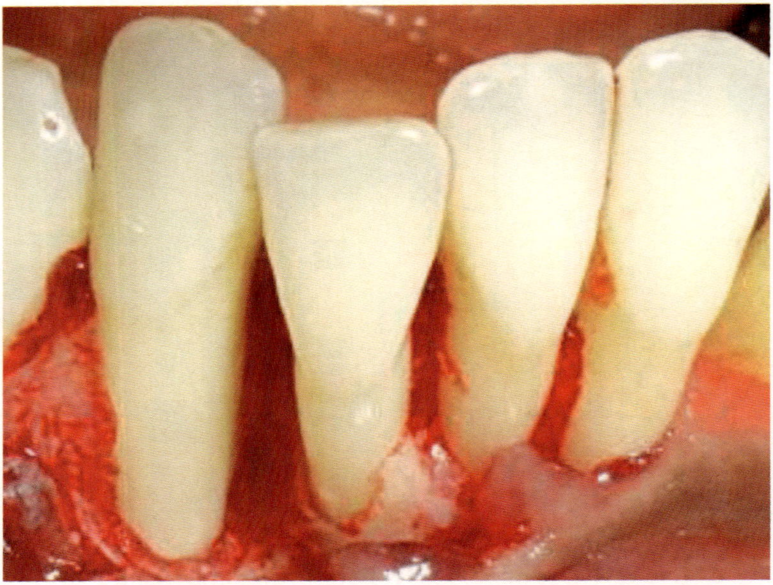

Fig. 8.2: Bony dehiscence and fenestration in lower anterior

Note: *Bone loss is often a combination of vertical and horizontal bone loss. Osseous surgery is the most predictable pocket reduction technique.*

Goal/Rationale of Osseous Resective Surgery

1. Reshape the marginal bone to resemble alveolar process undamaged by periodontal disease.
2. To eliminate periodontal pocket depth.
3. To improve tissue contour to provide a maintainable environment.

Terminologies (Fig. 8.3)

1. *Ideal osseous architecture:* Bone is more coronal on Interproximal surfaces than on facial and lingual surfaces.
2. *Positive architecture:* Radicular bone is apical to interdental bone.
3. *Negative architecture:* Interdental bone is apical than radicular bone.
4. *Flat architecture:* Reduction of interdental bone to the same height as radicular bone.

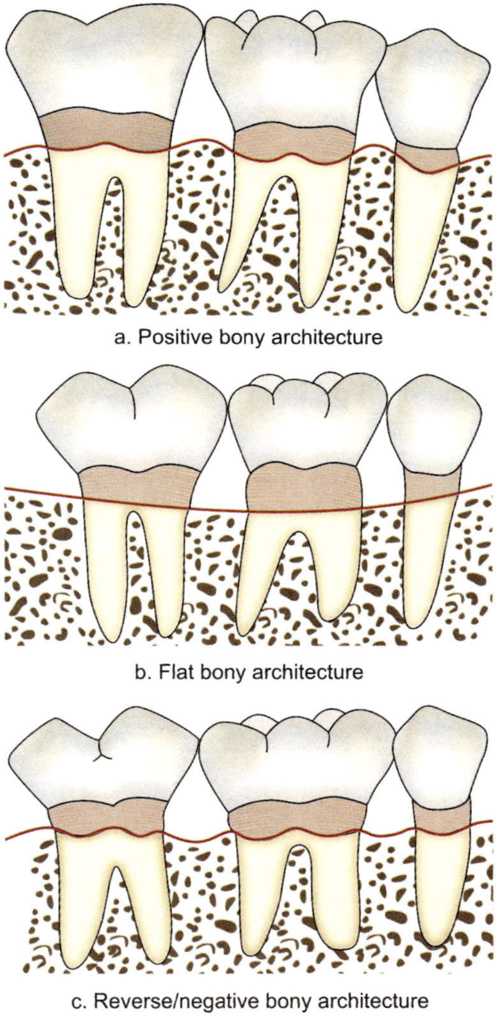

Fig. 8.3: Various types of bony architecture

Clinical Note

Transgingival probing/sounding of bone: *This technique is done under local anesthesia to confirm extent and configuration of intrabony component of pocket or furcation defects. Probe is "walked" along the tissue–tooth interface, to feel the bony topography.*

Osteoplasty

The purpose of osteoplasty is to create a physiologic form of the alveolar bone without removing any supporting bone.

Indications of Osteoplasty

1. Tori reduction, ledges
2. Shallow, blunted craters
3. Shallow buccal/lingual intrabony defects
4. Deep interproximal defects to achieve physiological contour
5. Proper approximation of flaps
6. Incipient furcation involvement
7. To provide space for pontic

Contraindications

1. Very thin bone and excessive resorption may occur.
2. If alternative therapy is available.

Ostectomy

In ostectomy, supporting bone, i.e. bone directly involved in the attachment of the tooth, is removed to reshape deformities caused by periodontitis in the marginal and interdental bone.

Indications of Ostectomy

1. Early to moderate bone loss (2–3 mm) with moderate length root trunks.
2. Intrabony defects not amenable to regenerative therapy in non-esthetic zones
3. Inconsistent bony margins
4. Moderate and advanced furcation involvement
5. Shallow to moderate craters
6. Hemiseptum
7. Crown lengthening/to expose subgingival caries

Contraindications

1. Insufficient remaining attachment, deep multiwalled defects
2. Anatomical limitations
3. Esthetic zones
4. Alternative treatment

Osseous Resection Technique

a. Vertical grooving
b. Radicular blending → Osteoplasty
c. Flattening interproximal bone
d. Gradualizing marginal bone → Ostectomy

Healing after osseous resective surgery is completed in 14–21 days.

Disadvantages of Resective Surgery

1. Causes recession and hypersensitivity, mostly in anterior and thin biotype.
2. Reduces tooth bone support.
3. Removes bone that may be needed, if implants are desired.
4. Exposed roots could be at higher risk for caries in patients with poor OHI. More access for brush but more challenge for patient to maintain.

Instrumentation in Resective Surgery

Freidman rongeurs, carbide round burs, diamond burs, interproximal files, back action chisels, Ochsenbein Chisel.

Craters (Fig. 8.4)

Craters are two-walled defects that occur at the expense of the interseptal bone. These are the most common bony defects in patients with periodontitis.

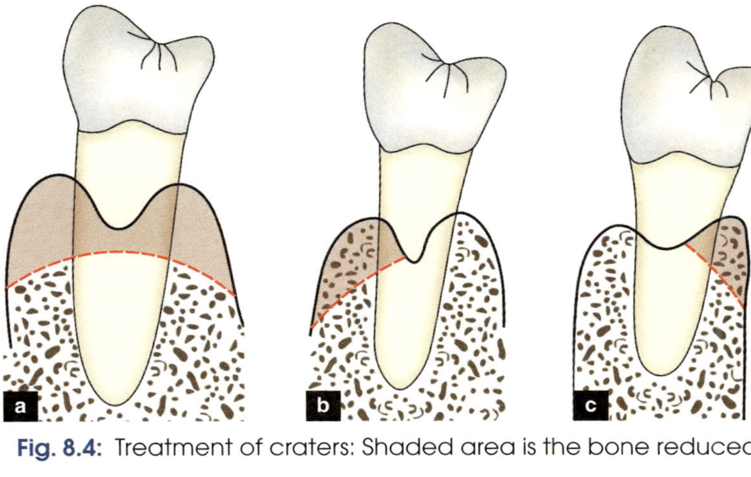

Fig. 8.4: Treatment of craters: Shaded area is the bone reduced

Craters are classified as

1. *Shallow:* 1–2 mm
2. *Medium:* 3–4 mm
3. *Deep:* 5 mm or more

Clinical Note (Fig. 8.5)

Widow's peaks: Peaks of bone left at facial and lingual/palatal line angles of the teeth after osteoplasty.

Treatment of Craters

a. Shallow to medium craters are treated with resective surgery.
b. Regenerative procedures can be aimed in deep craters.

The walls of craters may be reduced by:

1. Turning concavity into convexity: Reducing both facial and lingual walls.
2. At the expense of facial or lingual walls.

Ochsenbein and Bohannan,1964: Selective reduction of the bony defects in craters can be done by ramping the bone to the palatal/lingual wall. Selective reduction is indicated to achieve:

i. A satisfactory form
ii. Prevent therapeutic invasion of furcations
iii. Blend the contours with adjacent teeth

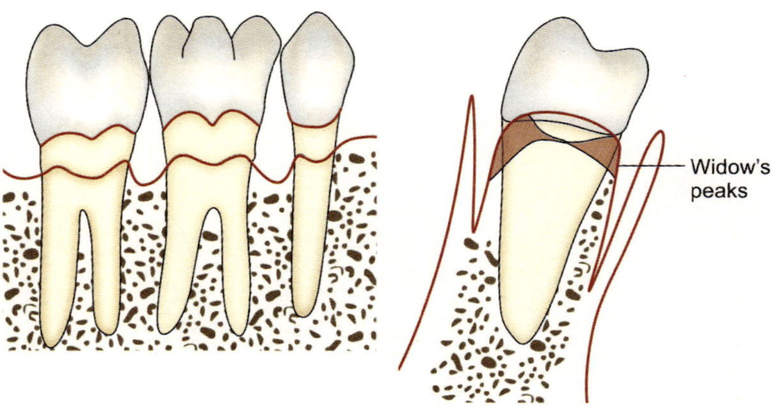

Fig. 8.5: Osteoplasty at line angles can result in widow's peaks

Author's Note

a. *Determination of bone defect morphology/type with clinical and radiographic tools is of utmost importance for planning the type of surgery respective or regenerative. A lot of time should be devoted in understanding the type of defects.*

b. *The objective of bone surgery is to establish a "physiologic" anatomy of the alveolar bone, but at a more apical level.*

c. *Care should be taken while doing ostectomy, not to create discrepancies of bone buccally/lingually or in interdental bone.*

d. *Osseous surgery should always be done under continuous saline irrigation to prevent bone necrosis.*

e. *Postoperative plaque control is the most important determinant of successful periodontal therapy.*

f. *Deep defects should be treated by a combination of resective and regenerative surgical procedures.*

Various Kinds of Defects (Fig. 8.6a to d)

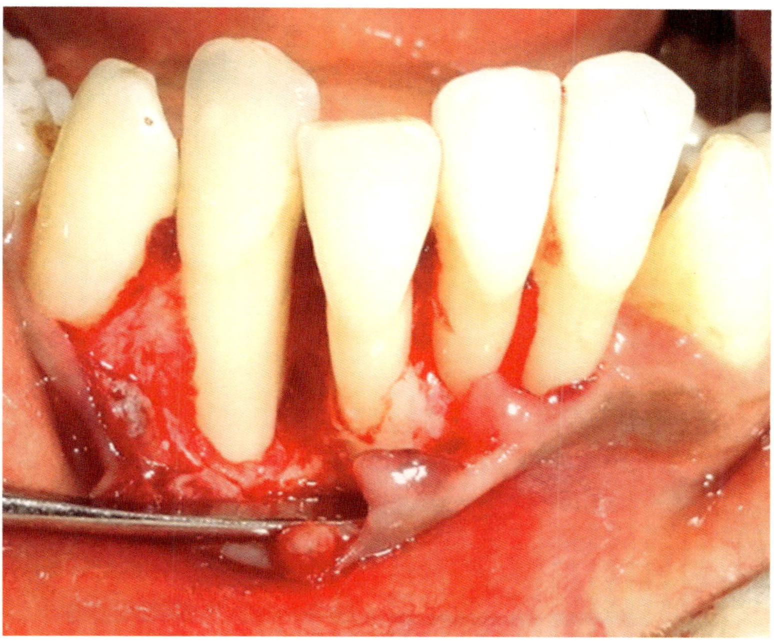

Fig. 8.6a: Two-walled vertical defect

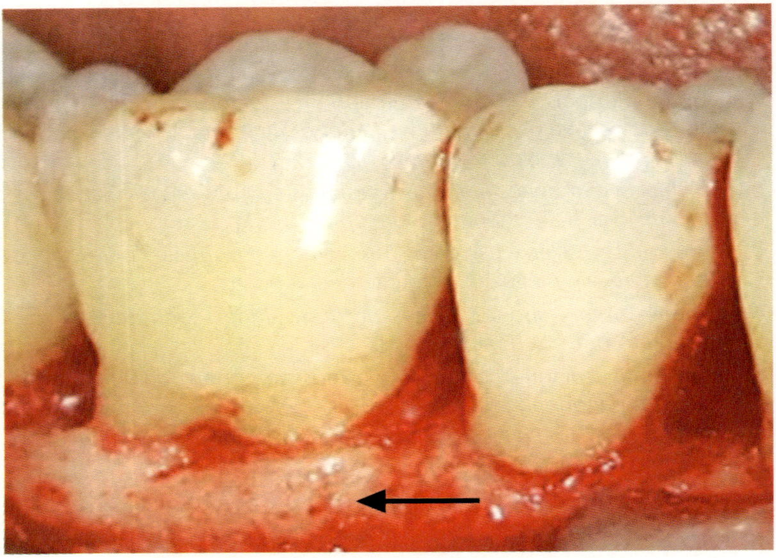

Fig. 8.6b: Bulbous bony margins

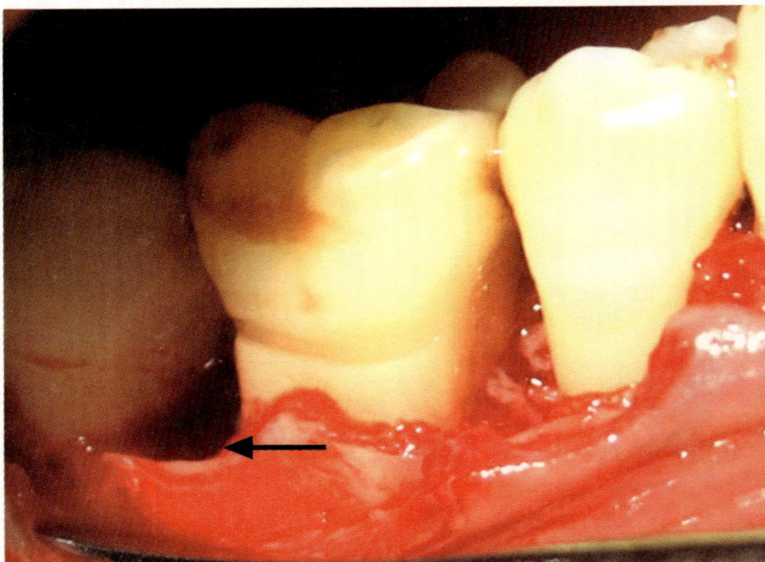

Fig. 8.6c: Ledges

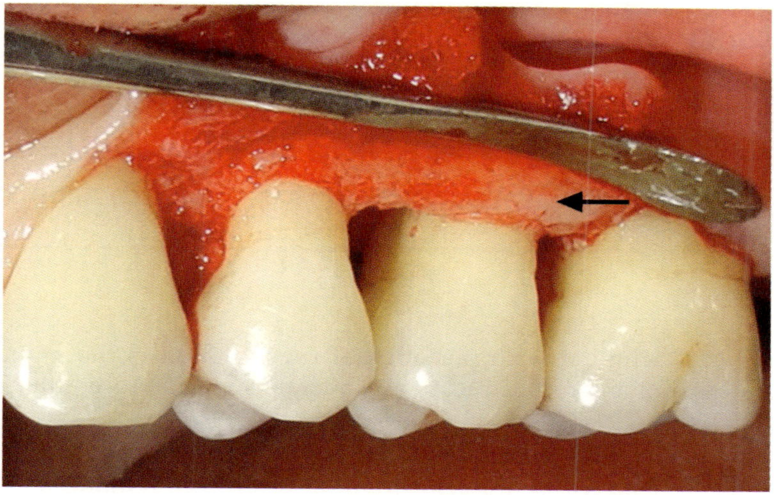

Fig. 8.6d: Exostoses

9 Reconstructive Periodontal Surgery

New attachment with periodontal regeneration is the main outcome of any reconstructive periodontal surgical procedure.

FEW TERMINOLOGIES

a. *Periodontal regeneration:* Restoration of lost periodontium or supporting tissues by regeneration includes formation of new alveolar bone, new cementum and new periodontal ligament.
b. *Repair:* Healing of a wound by a tissue that does not fully restore the architecture or function of the part. In periodontal repair, healing occurs by long junctional epithelium or epithelial adaptation or ankylosis.
c. *New attachment:* Union of connective tissue or epithelium with a root surface that has been previously deprived of its original attachment apparatus.
d. *Reattachment:* Reunion of epithelial and connective tissue with a previously healthy root surface after trauma or after supracrestal fibrotomy.
e. *Bone fill:* Clinical restoration of bone tissue in a treated periodontal defect.

CLASSIFICATION OF PROCEDURES

The procedures to achieve regeneration can be classified as below.

A. Non-Bone Graft Associated Procedures

1. Removal of junctional and pocket epithelium: Curettage, chemical agents (sodium sulfide, camphor, sodium hypochlorite), excisional new attachment procedures.
2. Clot stabilization/wound protection and space creation with guided tissue regeneration.

3. Preventing/impeding epithelial migration by:
   a. Root submergence
   b. Total removal of interdental papilla and replacement with free autogenous graft obtained from palate
   c. Coronally displaced flap to increase the distance between epithelial wound edge and healing area.
4. Biomodification of root surface: With citric acid, tetracycline, fibronectin.

B. Bone Graft Associated Procedures

Graft: It refers to viable tissues that after removal from a donor site are implanted within a recipient tissue for restoration by repair or regeneration.

Clinical Note

Implant is a nonliving tissue, a material inserted or grafted into intact tissue of recipient.

Classification of Bone Grafts by Hyatt and Butler (1957)

a. *Autograft:* Tissue taken from one operative site and grafted in another operative site within the same individual.
b. *Homograft:* Tissue taken from one operative site in one individual and grafted in the operative site in another individual of the same species.
c. *Heterograft:* Tissue taken from the one individual and grafted into the operative site of another individual of the different species.
d. *Isograft:* Tissue grafted from inbred strains (animals).
e. *Syngensis grafts:* Tissue graft removed from blood-related relatives.
f. *Orthotopic graft:* Tissue grafted into an anatomical site normally occupied by that tissue, e.g. bone-to-bone, skin-to-skin.

Mechanism of Bone Grafting

Bone grafting is accomplished through osteogenesis, osteoinduction and osteoconduction

1. *Osteogenesis:* Formation and development of bone by osteocompetent cells, which is derived from or composed of tissue involved in the natural growth and repair of bone, and

can stimulate bone formation in soft tissues, e.g. autogenous bone.

2. *Osteoinduction (Urist and Mclean, 1952):* It is the process of activating osteogenesis by recruiting cells from surrounding natural bone, then differentiate into bone forming cells, e.g. DFDBA.
3. *Osteoconduction* **(*Trellis's function*,** *Urist and colleagues, 1958):* It is also referred to as healing by creeping substitution. It is the process by which the graft material acts as a nonviable scaffold onto and within which the patients own natural bone grows. They allow apposition from existing bone, but do not produce or trigger bone formation, e.g. all alloplastic material.
4. *Osteopromotion:* Refers to the use of physical means to seal of an anatomical site, i.e. the site where bone is intended to be formed in order to prevent other tissues notably connective tissue, to interfere with osteogenesis.
5. *Osteotrophism:* Defined as an implantable matrix that provides improvement of bone formation by its chemical of structural characteristics in the presence of osteogenic precursor cells, e.g. natural bovine-derived HA.
6. *Contact inhibition (Ellegard and colleagues, 1976):* The process by which graft material prevents the apical proliferation of the epithelium.

Bone Grafts used in Clinical Practice

1. **Bone from intraoral sites:** Osseous coagulum, bone blend, cancellous bone marrow transplants, bone swaging
   a. Osseous coagulum (Robinson, 1969): Bone dust coated with blood to form coagulum.
   b. Bone blend (Diem et al, 1972): Bone is removed from a predetermined site, triturated in the capsule to a plastic-like mass and packed in bone defects.
   c. Bone swaging (Ewan, 1965) also called *contiguous autogenous transplant* or *pedicle bone graft*. It consists of pushing the bone from an edentulous site adjacent to the defect, without fracturing the bone at the apex.
   d. Intraoral cancellous bone marrow transplants from sites like maxillary tuberosity, edentulous area, healing socket.

2. **Bone from extraoral sites**
   a. *Iliac autografts:* Iliac autografts are one type of bone grafts from extraoral sites.

b. *Allograft:* Uncalcified freeze-dried bone allograft (osteoconductive), demineralized freeze-dried bone allograft (osteoinductive). Experiments by Urist et al have established the osteogenic potential of DFDBA.

c. *Xenografts:* Calf bone (boplant), an organic bone (ox bone), kiel bone (calf or ox bone).

d. Newer xenografts commercially available—bio oss (purified bovine-derived xenografts—(BDX), bio oss collagen, osteograft, nuoss.

e. Pep gen 15: Enhanced form of bovine hydroxyapatite that contains short chain peptide, P-15. Mimics the cell binding domain of type I collagen, which is responsible for cell migration, differentiation and proliferation.

3. **Bone substitutes**
   a. Xenogenic graft: Bovine derived, coral derived
   b. Alloplastic material: Polymers, bioceramics (tricalcium phosphate, hydroxyapatite), bioactive glasses and others
   c. Hard tissue replacement polymer (HTR polymer)—microporous, biocompatible composite of PMMA, PHEMA and calcium hydroxide
   d. Bioactive glass—contains sodium and calcium salts, phosphates and silicon dioxide. Available as perioglass (90–170 microns) and bioglass (300–355 microns)

Various New Materials Employed for Tissue Regeneration

1. Biological mediators—growth factors like insulin-derived growth factor, platelet-derived growth factor, recombinant human-derived growth factor (GEM-21S), bone morphogenetic proteins (BMP-2, BMP-7).
2. Enamel matrix proteins—mainly amelogenin secreted by Hertwig epithelial root sheath induces acellular cementum formation. Marketed under the name of Emdogain.

Surgical Procedure in Bone Grafting

I. *Criteria for selection of osseous graft (Schallhorn RG, 1977):*

a. Biologic acceptability

b. Predictability

c. Clinical feasibility

d. Minimum postoperative hazards
e. Patient acceptance

II. *Indications for bone grafting (Mellonig, 1982; Lynch, 2000)*

a. Three-walled/two-walled intrabony defect (deep narrow defects—ideal), deep craters.
b. Combined defect—three-walled at the apical and one-/two-walled defect at the coronal end, one-walled defect adjacent to edentulous area (bone swaging).
c. Furcation grade II and early grade III
d. Ridge augmentation, socket preservation, implant dentistry.
e. Increased bone support for a tooth.

III. *Type of flap-papilla preservation flap to achieve complete coverage for bone grafts*

IV. *Type of suturing with bone grafts—vertical mattress or intrapapillary. Ideally using monofilament—gore tex or vicryl suture*

V. *Assessment of clinical outcome*

Clinical criteria: Probing depth, attachment gain

PERIODONTAL REGENERATION—CLINICAL FACTS (POLSON)

A. Wound Healing

It has been Categorized into three Phases (Polson and Proye,1983):

1. Inflammation
2. Fibroblastic—granulation
3. Matrix formation and remodeling

At day 1: Fibrin clot adhesion to root surface.

At day 3: Long junctional epithelium formation after disruption of fibrin clot.

Clinical Note

Fibrin linkage and its adhesion to root surface is an important requisite to prevent formation of long junctional epithelium. Clinically, it is important to attain a close adaptation of the flap to the root surface and bone by suturing to promote periodontal regeneration.

B. Biological Considerations to Achieve Periodontal Regeneration

1. *Root surface alterations:* Normal root is rich in collagen and fibers, which gets destroyed by periodontitis.

A critical step in regenerative therapy is to alter periodontitis affected root surface to encourage epithelial migration, proliferation and increased migration of connective tissue progenitor cells.

Clinical Note

Root surface alteration can be done by thorough scaling and root planing, smearing with citric acid/EDTA, application of attachment proteins and growth factors.

2. *Epithelial exclusion:* Long junctional epithelium prevents regenerative therapy.

Clinical Note

Positioning the flap coronally, using GTR membranes, root submergence and are techniques to promote epithelial cell inclusion.

3. *Wound stabilization:* Early clot stabilization prevents epithelial downgrowth and forms a scaffold for collagen fiber attachment.

Clinical Note

Bone augmentation procedures and effective flap management contribute to wound stabilization.

4. *Reduced periodontium:* Periodontitis destroys the coronal periodontium. Bone augmentation grafts increase the height of attachment apparatus.

C. Bone Graft Technique

1. *Removal of etiologic factors:* Local and systemic factors should be removed for optimal success of bone graft surgery.
2. *Stabilization of teeth, if necessary:* Teeth with mobility should be stabilized pre- and postsurgically to achieve better occlusion and graft stability.
3. *Appropriate flap design:* Internal bevel, full thickness flap reflected beyond mucogingival junction, vertical incisions are recommended to allow proper access to defects and close the site at completion of surgery.
4. *Degranulation of defect and flap:* All granulomatous soft tissue, tissue tags on inner aspect of flap and epithelial remnants should be removed.
5. *Preparation of root:* Root surface alteration should be done to make a biologically acceptable root surface.
6. *Promotion of bleeding bony surface:* Intramarrow penetration with small round bur should be done to encourage bleeding and allow the ingress of reparative cells at defect site.
7. *Presuturing:* Loose placement of sutures, left untied, prior to filling of defect reduces the chances of displacement of graft while suturing.
8. *Adequate condensation of graft material:* The graft material should be placed in small increments with curettes/carriers/pluggers and condensed at defect site.
9. *Filling to a realistic level:* Overfilling should not be done as it interferes with proper flap closure, retards healing and also results in loss of graft material.
10. *Good tissue coverage:* Primary flap closure and contact of interproximal papillae should be achieved to cover bone graft site.

11. *Placement of periodontal dressing:* Firm, protective periodontal dressing for 10–14 days at defect site after bone graft surgery is recommended. Use of periodontal dressing after other periodontal procedures is controversial.
12. *Administration of antibiotics:* Administration of antibiotics after placement of bone grafts is recommended at least for 7 days to prevent immediate postsurgical inflammation and infection.
13. *Postsurgical care:* Thorough plaque control method by antibacterial rinses and professional check up by dentists is recommended.

Clinical Note

Grafted area should not be probed for 3 months postsurgically. Radiographs to check for bone fill should be taken at 6 months.

ADDITIONAL INFORMATION ON PERIODONTAL REGENERATION FOR POSTGRADUATES

1. Periodontal regeneration is possible even if a bone graft is not used as long as epithelial exclusion can be achieved.
2. Ideal indications of a bone graft are space maintenance, retain the blood clot, and serve as a scaffold to allow cell migration. Serve as an osteogenic matrix to allow differentiation of cells into osteoblasts.
3. There is histologic evidence of new bone formation and connective tissue attachment with bone grafts.
4. Guided tissue regeneration (GTR) favors a new connective tissue attachment with or without new bone formation.

   Classical study for the importance of periodontal ligament cells in regenerative procedures—Loe and Waerhaug, 1961.
5. Wide shallow defects heal faster than deep narrow defects. Critical phase of healing occurs within first 2 months.

   Aukhil et al, 1988: Periodontal ligament cells migrate at a short distance with or without a physical barrier. The critical role of a membrane is to allow migrant cells sufficient time for population of root surface.
6. Till date, cortical DFDBA is considered an ideal bone graft that has proven to stimulate bone formation.
7. ***Nyman et al, 1982, Karring et al, 1980, Gottlow et al, 1984- Classical studies on bone regeneration.***

Regenerative Therapy in Grade II Furcation

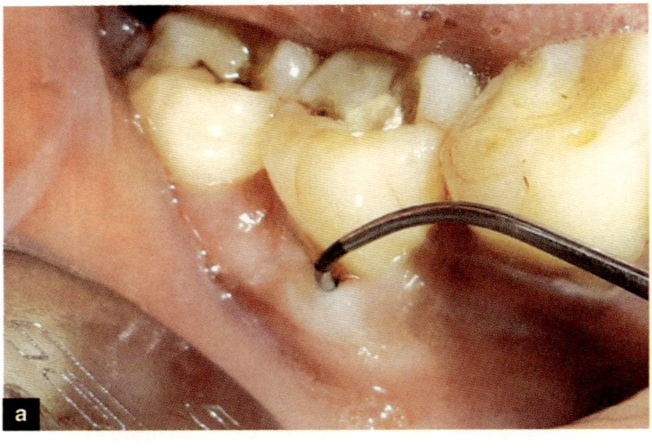
a

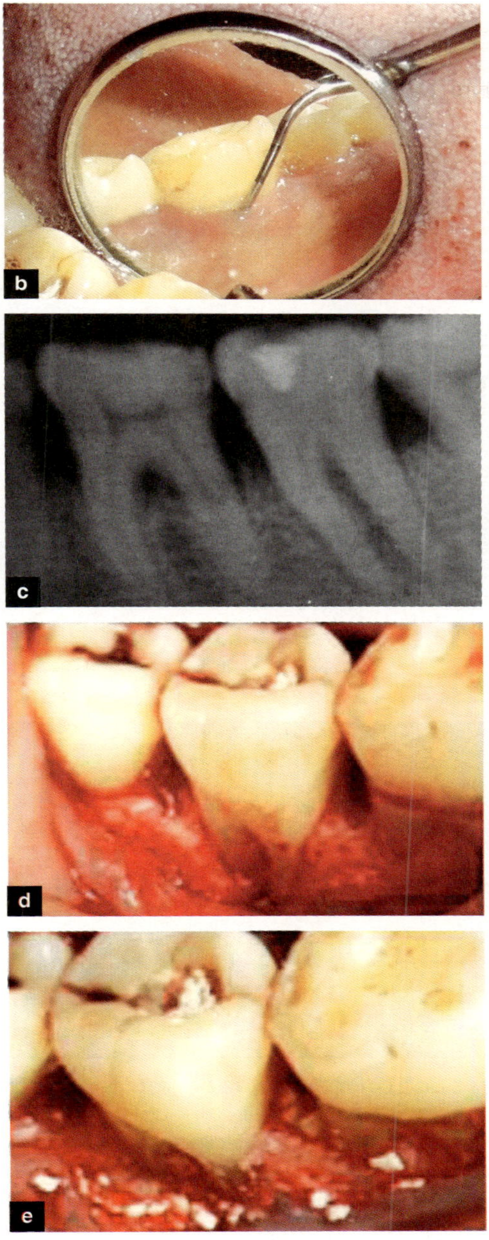
b
c
d
e

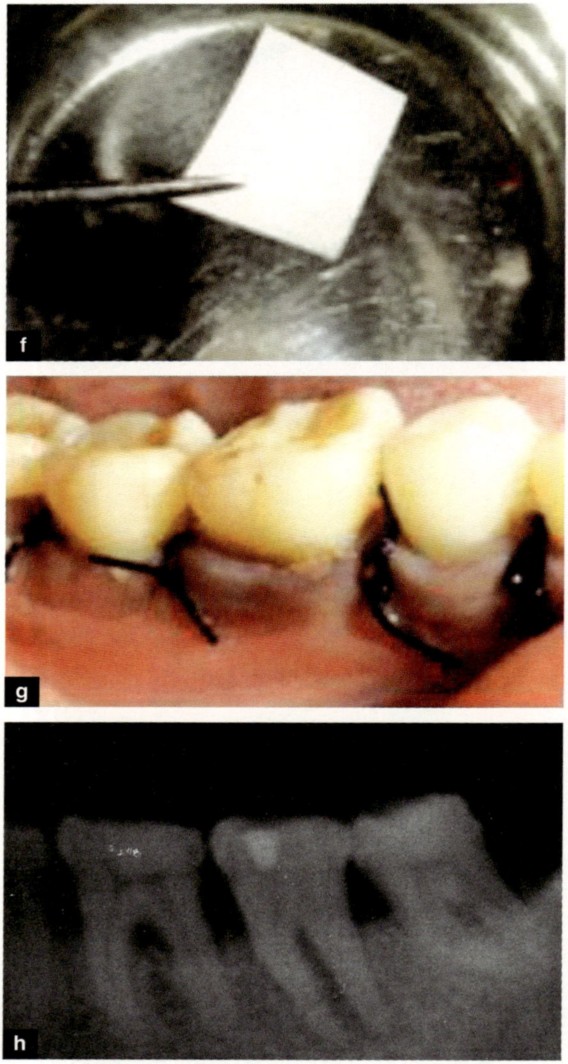

Fig. 9.1a to h: (a and b) Preoperative horizontal component of grade II furcation 47 buccally—9 mm and lingually—6 mm. Probing with noncoded Nabers' probe; (c) IOPA shows advanced bone loss; (d and e) Kirkland flap raised and debridement done; (f) Calcium hydroxy-apetite and collagen membrane placed; (g) Flaps adapted and sutured; (h) After 3 months, bone fill can be observed

10

Furcation—Diagnosis and Treatment

A furcation is defined as the anatomic area of a multirooted tooth where the roots diverge (Fig. 10.1).

Furcation invasion refers to pathologic resorption of bone within a furcation.

Classification of Furcation Involvement

1. Glickmans (1953) classification

Grade I

1. Incipient or early stage
2. Soft-tissue lesion or pocket extending into flute of furcation
3. Suprabony pocket

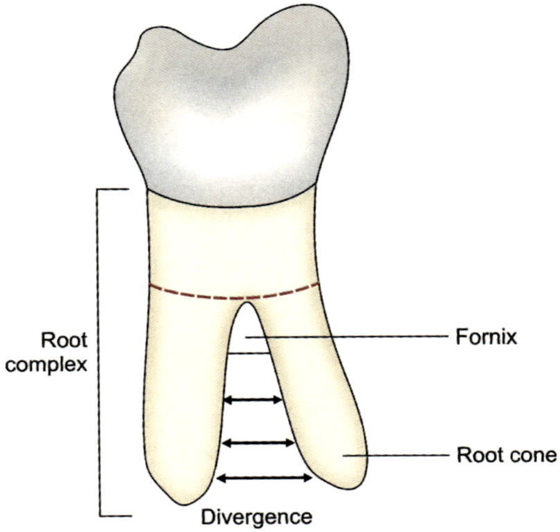

Fig. 10.1: Root anatomy

4. Inter-radicular bone → intact or slight bone loss
5. Radiographic evidence of bone loss is usually not there

Grade II

1. Pocket formation and loss of inter-radicular bone of varying depths into the furcation but not through and through.
2. Portion of PDL and bone remains intact.
3. Cul de sac with a horizontal component
4. Partial penetration of probe
5. Radiographs may or may not depict involvement especially in maxillary molars.

Grade III

1. Complete loss of inter-radicular bone
2. Radiographic evidence of small triangular radiolucency
3. Periodontal pocket is completely probable to the opposite side of the tooth.
4. Furcation not visible clinically. It is occluded by gingival tissue.

Grade IV

Same as Grade III except that loss of periodontal attachment and gingival recession. Furcation is clearly visible on a clinical examination.

2. Goldmans classification: Classified as incipient, cul de sac and complete.

3. Hamp, Nyman and Lindhe (1975)

Class I: Horizontal attachment loss of <3 mm within the furcation involvement (not exceeding 1/3rd width of tooth).

Class II: Horizontal loss greater than 3 mm (exceeding 1/3rd width of tooth) but not encompassing the total width of the furcation.

Class III: Horizontal through and through destruction of periodontal tissues in the furcation area.

4. Tarnow and Fletcher (1984)

Subclass A: Vertical destruction to one-third of the total inter-radicular height (3 mm or less).

Subclass B: Vertical destruction reaching two-thirds of the inter-radicular height (4 to 6 mm).

Subclass C: Inter-radicular osseous destruction into or beyond the apical third (>7 mm).

5. Fedi (1985)

a. Combined Glickman and Hamp Classification
b. Same Glickman's Grade I to Grade IV

Grade II subdivided into:
- *Degree I:* Less than 3 mm involvement
- *Degree II:* More than 3 mm involvement

Cervical Enamel Projections (Masters and Hoskins, 1964)

CEPs are present in more than 90% of furcation involvements in mandibular molars.

Grade 1: Enamel projection extend from the CEJ of tooth towards furcation entrance

Grade 2: Enamel projection approaches the entrance to furcation. Does not enter the furcation so no horizontal component.

Grade 3: Enamel projection extends horizontally into furcation.

Clinical Note

In maxillary molars, distal furcation is located midway buccolingually, hence probing from both sides. Mesial furcations are located 2/3rds towards palate, hence probed from palatal aspect.

Probing Methods

a. Probing done with curved graduated periodontal probe
b. An explorer
c. A small curette
d. Nabers probe (coded and noncoded).

Recommended Methods of Furcation Therapy (Lindhe, 1988)

Degree I: SRP, furcationplasty

Degree II: Furcationplasty, GTR at mandibular molars, tunnel preparation, root resection

Degree III: Tunnel preparation, root resection, tooth extraction

Root Resection

Indications for Root Resection

1. Indicated in grade II to grade IV furcations: Severe bone loss affecting one or more roots untreatable with regenerative procedures, Class II or Class III furcation invasions, severe recession or dehiscence of a root.

2. Inability to successfully treat and fill a canal, root fracture or root perforation, severe root resorption, root decay.
3. Severe root proximity inadequate for a proper embrasure space, root trunk fracture or decay with invasion of the biological width.

Which Root to Remove in Root Resection? (Fig. 10.2)

1. Remove the root that eliminates the furcation.
2. The root with maximum amount of bone and attachment loss.
3. Remove the root, removal of which eliminated periodontal problem on adjacent teeth.
4. Root with greater amount of anatomical problems.
5. Remove the root, removal of which least complicates periodontal maintenance.

Laser Therapy in Furcation Treatment

Er:YAG laser has been tried in treatment of grade III furcation defects. The results showed new bone formation at the site at 3 months.

Recent Treatment Concepts

1. Periodontal ligament cells in tissue engineering with GTR
2. Topical application of rhβ-MP2 and rh β-NGF

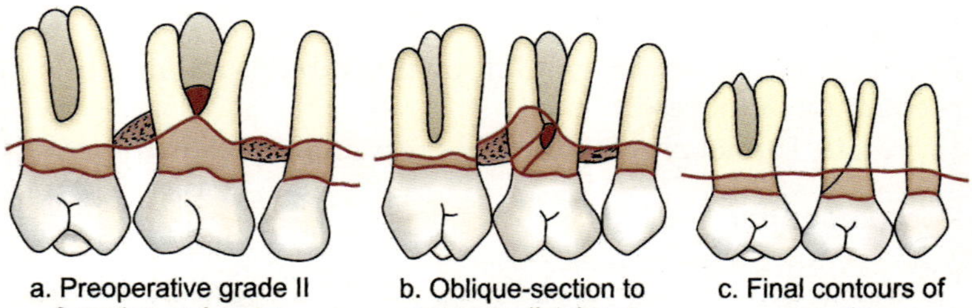

a. Preoperative grade II furcation and crater between first and second molars

b. Oblique-section to separate distal root

c. Final contours of resection

Fig. 10.2: Sequence of steps in root resection

Root Resection (Figs 10.3 to 10.8)

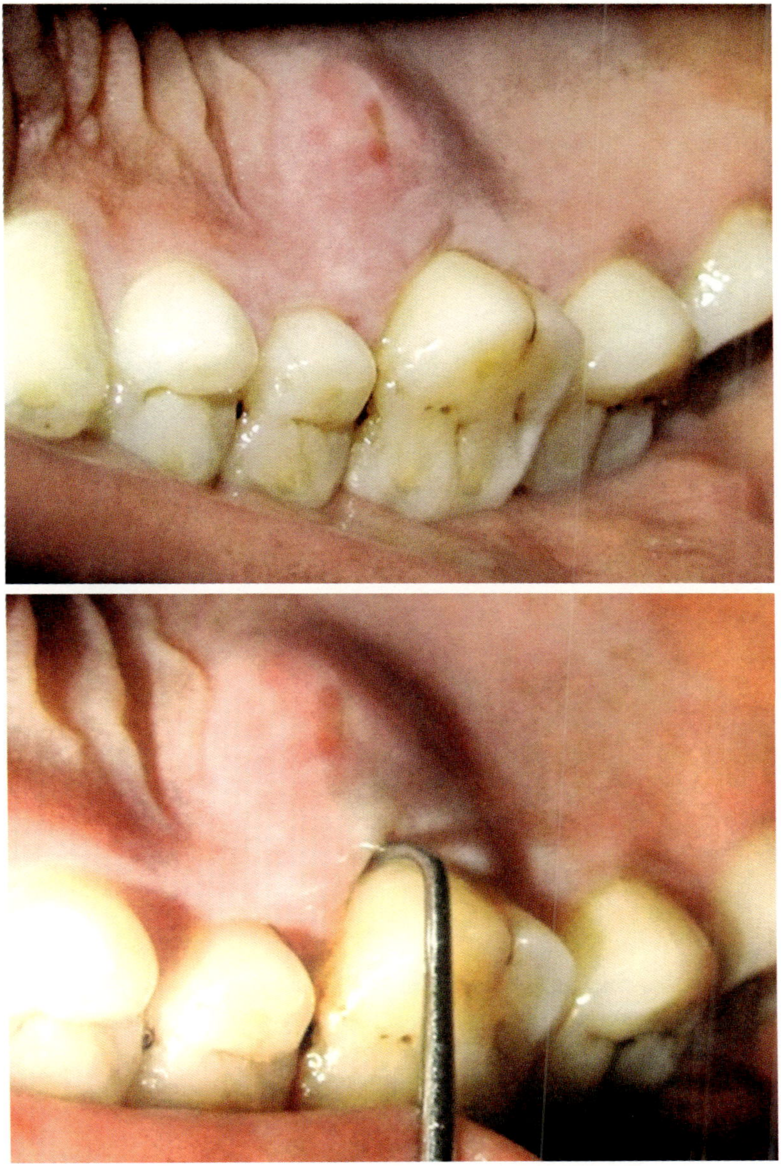

Fig. 10.3: Palatal abscess 16 with pocket probing depth of 10 mm

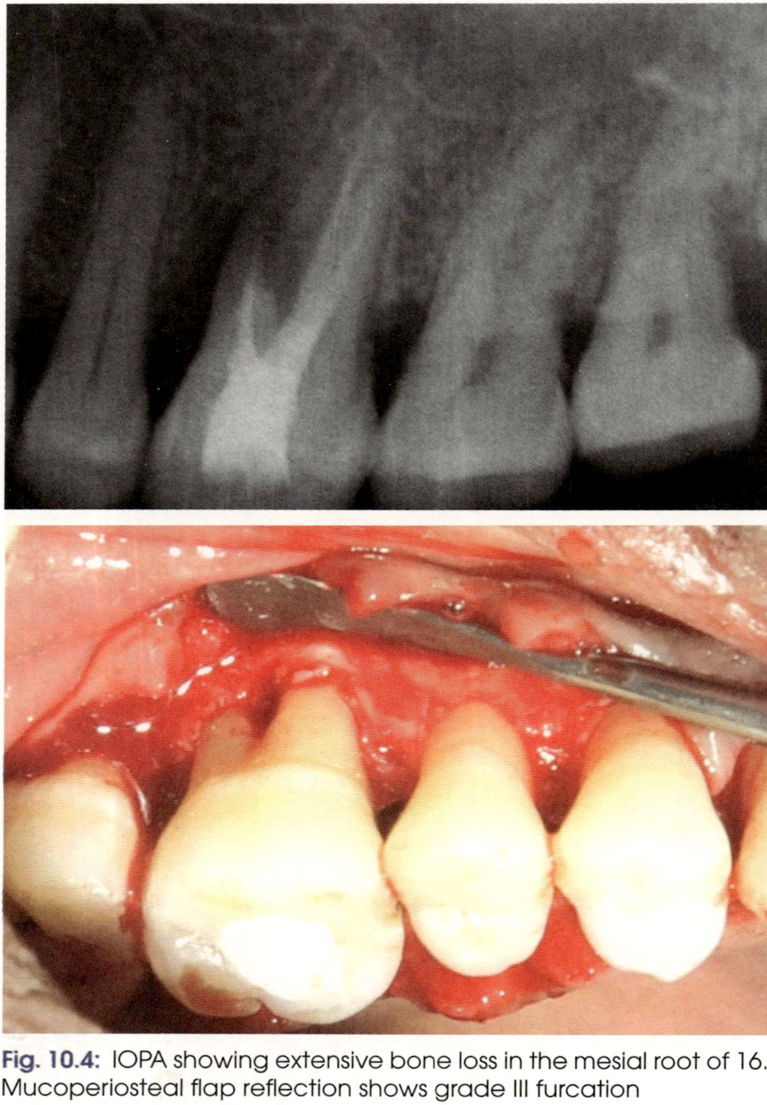

Fig. 10.4: IOPA showing extensive bone loss in the mesial root of 16. Mucoperiosteal flap reflection shows grade III furcation

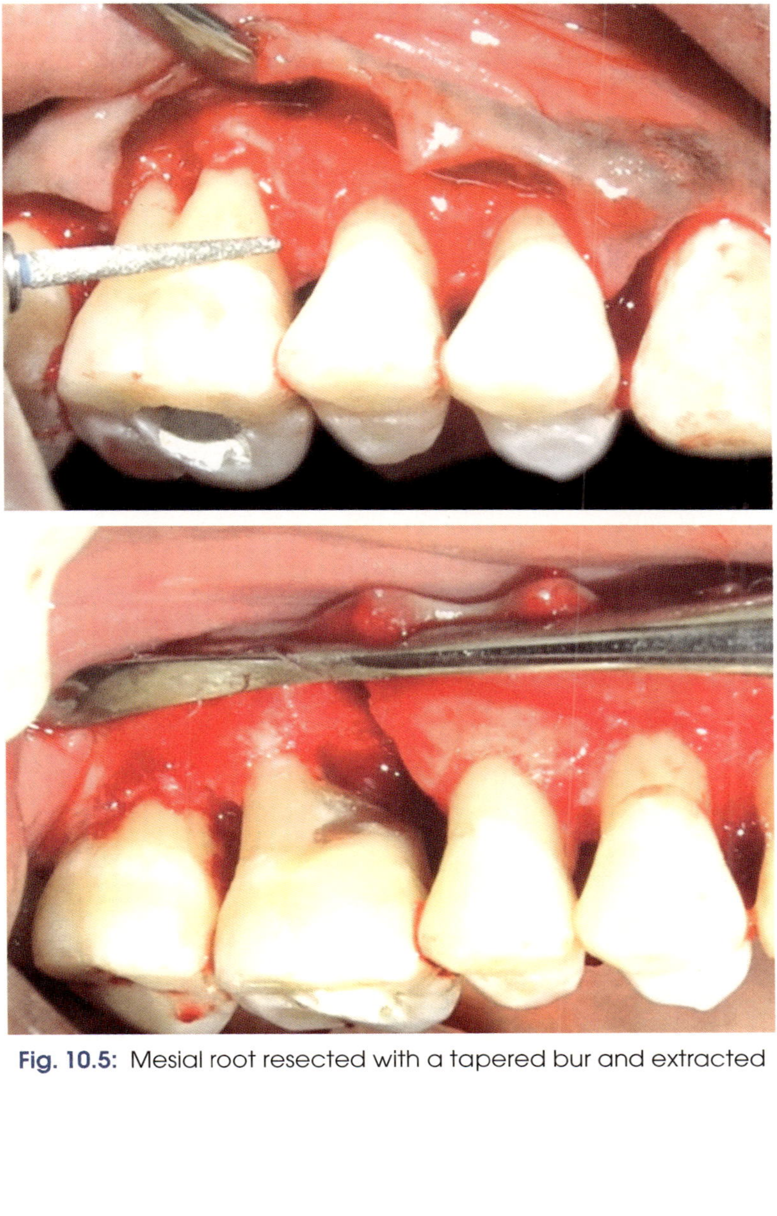

Fig. 10.5: Mesial root resected with a tapered bur and extracted

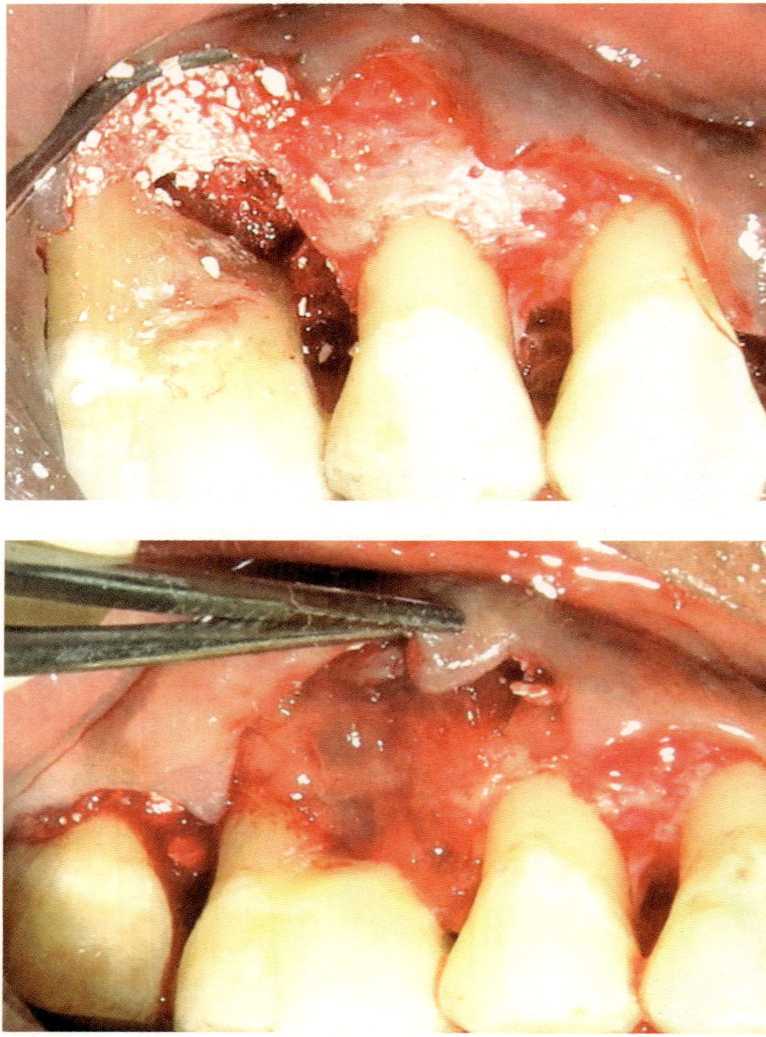

Fig. 10.6: Bone graft placed along with PRF placed as a barrier

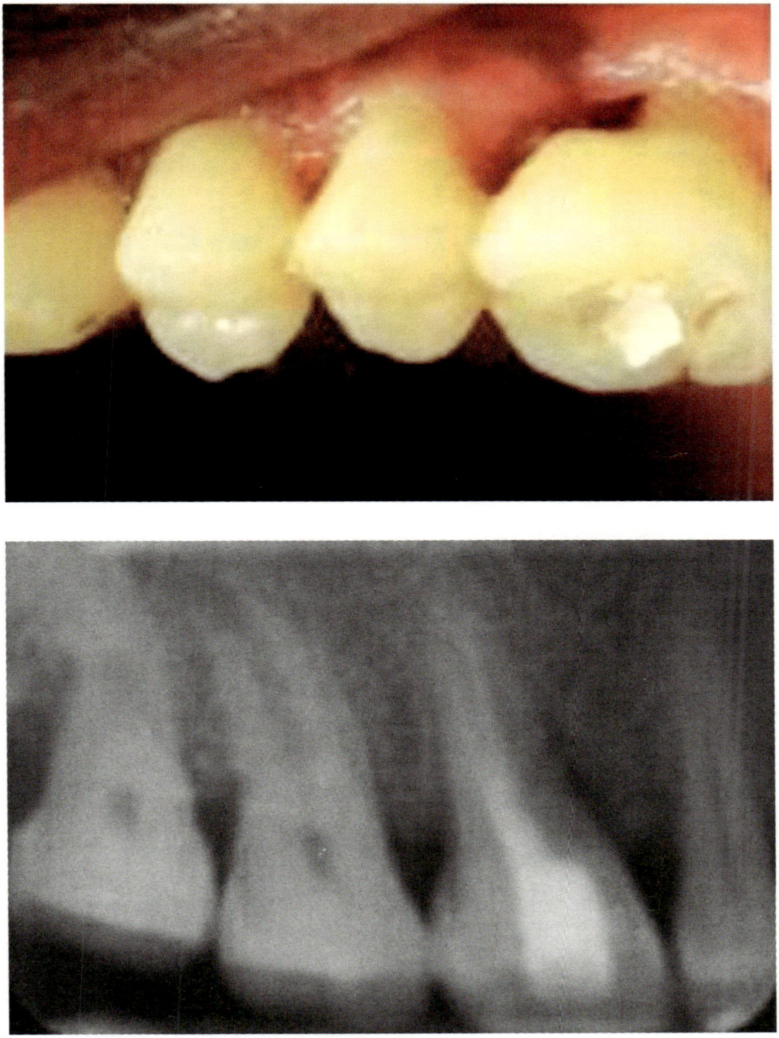

Fig. 10.7: Postoperative after 3 months

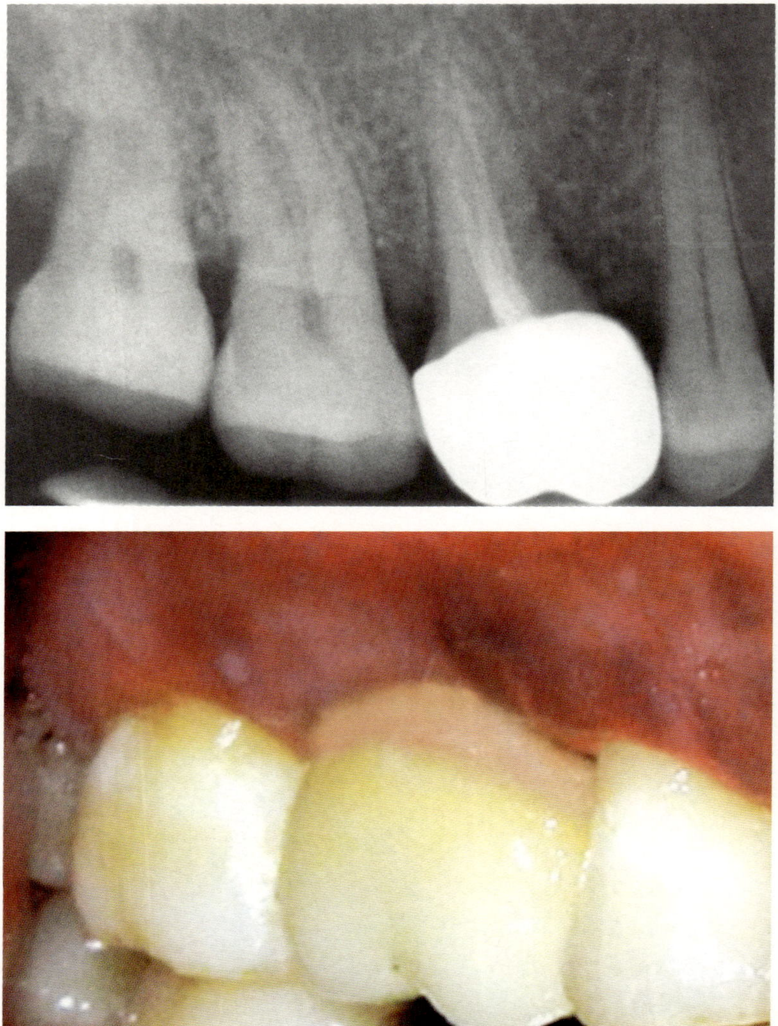

Fig. 10.8: Postoperative after crown cementation

11

Gingival Recession

Gingival recession is defined as the displacement of marginal tissue apical to the CEJ with the denudation of the root surface (glossary of periodontal terms, 2001).

Note: *Recession is a finding; mucogingival problem is a diagnosis.*

Pure Mucogingival Problem

Pure mucogingival problems are caused by a tooth erupting in prominence at or near the mucogingival junction so that little or no attached gingiva is present over the prominent root of the fully erupted (Hall, 1984).

Etiology

Traumatizing toothbrushing and tooth malpositioning are most frequently found to be associated with gingival recession.

Classification of Etiology of Gingival Recession (Hall et al, 1977)

Predisposing Factors

1. Inadequate attached gingiva
2. High frenal attachment
3. Malpositioning of teeth
4. Osseous dehiscence

Precipitating Factors

1. Improper brushing technique
2. Presence of plaque and resultant inflammation

3. Iatrogenic
4. Habits
5. TFO

Classification Systems for Gingival Recession

1. Sullivan and Atkins (1968)

a. Shallow narrow
b. Shallow wide
c. Deep narrow
d. Deep wide

2. Miller's classification, 1985 (Fig. 11.1)

It is a diagnostic and prognostic classification. Determines the level of root coverage achievable with a free gingival graft.

a. *Class I:* Marginal tissue recession which does not extend to the mucogingival junction (MGJ). There is no alveolar bone loss or soft tissue loss in the interdental area. Complete root coverage is obtainable.
b. *Class II:* Marginal tissue recession which extends to or beyond the MGJ. There is no alveolar bone loss or soft tissue loss in the interdental area. Complete root coverage is obtainable.
c. *Class III:* Marginal tissue recession which extends to or beyond the MGJ. Bone or soft tissue loss in the interdental area is present. Partial root coverage related to level of papilla height.
d. *Class IV:* Marginal tissue recession which extends to or beyond the MGJ. The bone or soft tissue loss in the interdental area is present with gross flattening. No root coverage obtainable.

3. Pinni Prato (2010)

Recession associated with abrasion defect:

Class a: CEJ seen

- + Step present
- – Step absent

Class b: CEJ not seen

- + Step present
- – Step absent

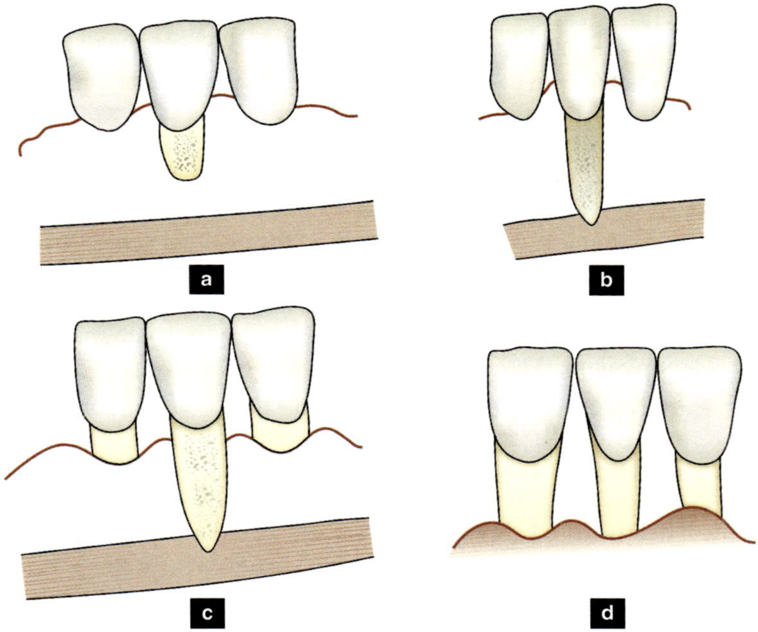

Fig. 11.1a to d: Miller's classification: (a) Class I; (b) Class II; (c) Class III; (d) Class IV. Complete loss of interdental papilla

4. Mahajan's modification of Miller's classification (2010)

a. *Class I:* Gingival recession defect (GRD) not extending to the mucogingival junction (MGJ).
b. *Class II:* GRD extending to the MGJ/beyond it.
c. *Class III:* GRD with bone or soft-tissue loss in the interdental area up to cervical one-third of the root surface and/or malpositioning of the teeth.
d. *Class IV:* GRD with severe bone or soft-tissue loss in the interdental area greater than cervical one-third of the root surface and/or severe malpositioning of the teeth.

Prognosis

a. *Best:* Class I and Class II with thick gingival profile.
b. *Good:* Class I and Class II with thin gingival profile.
c. *Fair:* Class III with thick gingival profile.
d. *Poor:* Class III and Class IV with thin gingival profile

5. **New classification system for gingival and palatal recession—Ashish Kumar and Sujata Surendra Masamatti (2013)**

   This classification can be applied for facial surfaces of maxillary teeth and facial and lingual surfaces of mandibular teeth.

   Class I: There is no loss of interdental bone or soft-tissue. This is subclassified into two categories:
   - *Class IA:* Gingival margin on F/L aspect lies apical to CEJ, but coronal to MGJ with attached gingiva present between marginal gingiva and MGJ.
   - *Class IB:* Gingival margin on F/L aspect lies at or apical to MGJ with an absence of attached gingiva between marginal gingiva and MGJ.

   Either of the subdivisions can be on facial or lingual aspect or both (F and L).

   Class II: The tip of the interdental papilla is located between the interdental contact point and the level of the CEJ mid-buccally/mid-lingually. Interproximal bone loss is visible on the radiograph. This is subclassified into three categories:
   - *Class IIA:* There is no marginal tissue recession on F/L aspect.
   - *Class IIB:* Gingival margin on F/L aspect lies apical to CEJ but coronal to MGJ with attached gingiva present between marginal gingiva and MGJ.
   - *Class IIC:* Gingival margin on F/L aspect lies at or apical to MGJ with an absence of attached gingiva between marginal gingiva and MGJ.

   Either of the subdivisions can be on F or L aspect or both (F and L).

   Class III: The tip of the interdental papilla is located at or apical to the level of the CEJ mid-buccally/mid-lingually. Interproximal bone loss is visible on the radiograph. This is subclassified into two categories:
   - *Class IIIA:* Gingival margin on F/L aspect lies apical to CEJ, but coronal to MGJ with attached gingiva present between marginal gingiva and MGJ.
   - *Class IIIB:* Gingival margin on F/L aspect lies at or apical to MGJ with an absence of attached gingiva between marginal gingiva and MGJ.

   Either of the subdivisions can be on F or L aspect or both (F and L)

6. **Classification of palatal gingival recession:** The position of interdental papilla remains the basis of classifying gingival recession on palatal aspect. The criteria of subclassifications have been modified to compensate for the absence of MGJ.

   PR-I deals with marginal tissue recession on palatal aspect with no loss of interdental bone or soft-tissue. This is subclassified into two categories:
   - *PR-IA:* Marginal tissue recession ≤3 mm from CEJ
   - *PR-IB:* Marginal tissue recession >3 mm from CEJ

   PR-II and PR-III deal with the loss of interdental bone/soft-tissue with marginal tissue recession on palatal aspect. This is subclassified into two categories:
   - *PR-IIA:* Marginal tissue recession ≤3 mm from CEJ
   - *PR-IIB:* Marginal tissue recession of >3 mm from CEJ

Palatal recession-III: The tip of the interdental papilla is located at or apical to the level of the CEJ mid-palatally. Interproximal bone loss is visible on the radiograph. This is subclassified into two categories:
- *PR-IIIA:* Marginal tissue recession ≤3 mm from CEJ
- *PR-IIIB:* Marginal tissue recession of >3 mm from CEJ

Classification of Root Coverage Procedures
(Wennstrom et al, 1996)

I. Pedicle grafts
   A. Rotational flaps
      a. Laterally positioned flap
      b. Obliquely rotated flap
      c. Double papilla flap
   B. Advanced flap
      a. Coronally positioned flap
      b. Semilunar coronally positioned flap

II. Free soft tissue graft
   A. Epithelialized soft tissue graft (classical gingival graft)
   B. Non-epithelialized soft tissue graft

III. Combination grafts.
   A. CT+ laterally positioned
   B. CT+ double papilla Nelson
   C. CT+ coronally positioned

D. Envelope technique and modification
E. Alloderm+ coronally positioned

IV. Additive treatment: Root biomodification, enamel matrix proteins, fibrin adhesive system, platelet rich plasma (PRP) and platelet rich fibrin (PRF).

Free Gingival Graft (FGG)/Epithelialized Palatal Graft (Bjorn, 1963)

Indications

1. To widen the zone of attached gingiva
2. To enable the patient practice good plaque control by creating a new zone of soft tissue.

Sullivan and Atkins classified free gingival graft thickness as:

a. Thin—less than 0. 5 mm
b. Intermediate—0.5 to 0.75 mm
c. Thick—1.25 to 2 mm

Variant of free gingival graft:

a. Accordion technique—Rateitschak, 1985
b. Strip technique—Han et al, 1993

Healing phases in FGG (Oliver et al, 1968)

a. Plasmatic circulation stage (2–3 days)
b. Capillary circulation stage (4–11 days)—revascularization begins
c. Tissue maturation stage (12–42 days)—organic union phase

Clinical Note for Technique

1. *The width of recipient site should be twice the desired width of attached gingiva to compensate for the contraction of graft that occurs during healing.*
2. *An aluminium foil can be used as a template for the graft size.*
3. *The graft to be harvested from the palate should be of intermediate thickness (1–1.5 mm)—**equivalent to width of the bevel on the** blade.*
4. *Graft can be placed directly on bone tissue also. This technique results in better hemostasis, less shrinkage of graft and less swelling.*
5. *There should not be any clot, tissue tags between the graft and recipient site as it impairs vascularization of graft. The graft should be immobilized, with no excessive tension by suturing.*
6. *Palatal site should be sutured, after bleeding is controlled by ice water, hemostats, pressure application. Pack should be placed and patient reviewed after a week.*

Note:

a. *Healing of graft of intermediate thickness completed by 10.5 weeks.*
b. *Healing of thicker graft completed by 16 weeks or longer*
c. *Healing phenomenon frequently observed following free graft procedures is* ***"Creeping attachment"—proposed by Goldman****. It is the coronal migration of the soft tissue margin. This occurs as consequence of tissue maturation during a period of about 1 year post-treatment.*

Connective Tissue Graft (Edel, 1974)

Rationale for use of connective tissue graft: Connective tissue bears the genetic information for the keratinization of overlying epithelium.

Advantages

1. Better color match, hence improved aesthetics.
2. Less postoperative discomfort to the patient and healing is by first intention.

Connective tissue technique—Levine, 1991.

Clinical Note for Technique

1. *Connective tissue is most commonly procured from the palate. Safe incision is from mesial line angle of the palatal root of first molar to distal line angle of the canine.*
2. *The neurovascular bundle may be located 7 to 17 mm from the cementoenamel junctions of the maxillary premolars and molars. Take precaution while extending the incision too wide.*

Distance of neurovascular bundle in average palate is 12 mm, 7 mm in shallow palate and 17 mm in high palate

3. *Incisions to harvest CT can be classified as (Liu classification) (Fig. 11.2):*
   a. *One incision or envelope incision*
   b. *Two incisions: L-shaped incision*
   c. *U-shaped or trap door incision*
4. *The graft should be kept immediately at recipient site or kept moist by keeping in saline after harvesting.*
5. *Thickness of graft, coronal repositioning of the flap, suturing are the factors determining the end result.*

Modifications of Connective Tissue Graft

1. Langer and Langer (1985)—Subepithelial connective tissue graft
2. Allen (1994)—Tunnel approach
3. Harris (1994)—Partial thickness pedicle graft with CTG
4. Nelson (1987)—Subpedicle connective tissue graft

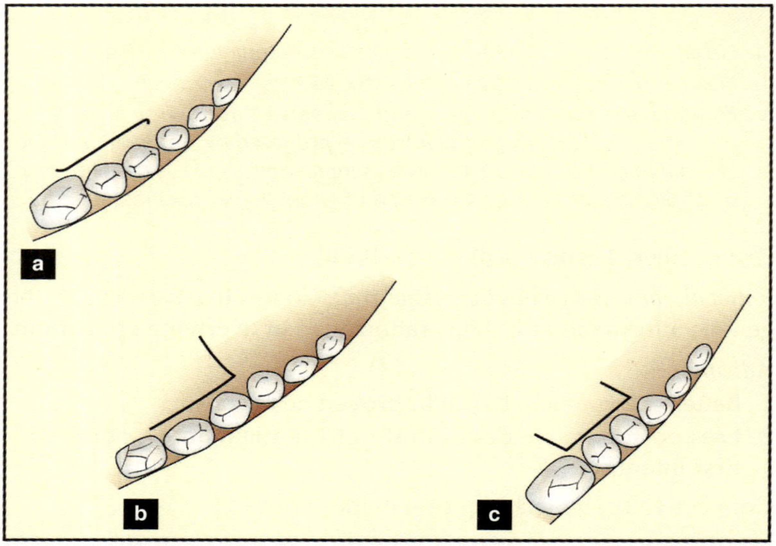

Fig. 11.2a and c: Various types of incisions: (a) Single incision; (b) Two incisions/L shaped; (c) Three incisions

Pedicle Autografts

I. Laterally displaced flap (Grupe and Warren, 1956)

Indications

1. To cover isolated, denuded root surfaces that have adequate adjacent donor tissue.
2. Presence of adequate vestibular depth.

Advantage: Good vascularity of the pedicle flap

Variant:

Modifications

1. *Periosteally stimulated pedicle flap by Smukler and Goldman (1978):* It is based on the rationale that stimulated periosteum activates primordial cells capable of bone and cementum. In this technique, periosteum is activated with a sharp instrument or 25 gauge needle used to make sharp penetrations through the gingiva 17 to 21 days prior to performing LPG.
2. *Double papilla graft by Cohen and Ross (1968):* Bilateral interdental papilla is used as a donor tissue low predictability of success.

Clinical Note for Technique

1. *Epithelium at the site of denuded root surface should be removed by scraping. It is done to expose the connective tissue which will make contact with the donor flap.*
2. *A partial or full thickness donor flap can be used. Its better to use a partial thickness flap as it reduces the risk of loss of facial bone height and also the healing time at the donor site. If the gingival biotype is thin, use a full thickness flap.*
3. *The flap should be sufficiently wide (almost by 11/2 times) to provide a broad attachment area.*
4. ***A cut back incision****—short oblique releasing incision at the distal corner of the flap in the direction of recipient site should be made to avoid tension at the base of the flap.*

Results are controversial since blood supply is compromised due to suturing at the mid-surface of root.

Healing of pedicle soft tissue grafts (Wilderman and Wentz, 1965)

a. The adaptation stage (from 0 to 4 days).
b. The proliferation stage (from 4 to 21 days).
c. The attachment stage (from 27 to 28 days).
d. The maturation stage.

Apically Displaced Flap

Friedman and Levin (1962) Classification

Class I

1. More than adequate keratinized gingival width
2. Labial or buccal incision 1–3 mm from crest of gingiva.
3. Flap apically positioned to cover 1–2 mm of cementum.

Class II

1. Adequate keratinized gingiva.
2. Crestal incision is used.
3. Flap apically positioned to the crest of the bone.

Class III

1. Insufficient gingival keratinized width.
2. Sulcular incision.
3. Flap is positioned 1–2 mm below crest of bone to increase the width of keratinized gingiva.

Clinical Note for Technique

1. *Indications of apically displaced flap are pocket eradication and increasing the width of attached gingiva.*
2. *An internal bevel incision directed at the crest of the bone is the first step. The incision is not related to the pocket depth.*
3. *In cases of crown lengthening, it is preferred over gingivectomy to prevent biologic width violation.*
4. *Suturing and stabilization of the flap is an important consideration.*

Coronally Advanced Flap Introduced by Norberg (1926)

Bernimoulin (1975) graphically outlined the procedure as it is practiced today.

Clinical Note for Technique

1. *There are two techniques: In the first technique, split thickness flap is raised with internal bevel incision and two vertical incisions.*
2. *Bernimoulin technique (1975) is a modification of first technique, which is a two-step procedure. Gingival augmentation with free gingival graft followed by coronally positioned flap.*
3. *Second technique—Semilunar coronally advanced flap by Tarnow (1986)*
4. *In semilunar flap, care should be taken to extend the incision 2–3 mm short of the tip of papillae. This technique does not involve suturing. Indicated mostly in maxilla, in areas where gingival recession is not more than 3 mm and gingival biotype is thick.*

Modification

1. Laterally moved, coronally advanced flap—Zuccheli et al, 2004 (Fig. 11.3)
   a. Indicated in teeth with multiple gingival recessions.
   b. Split-full-split thickness flap—helps in better coronal placement

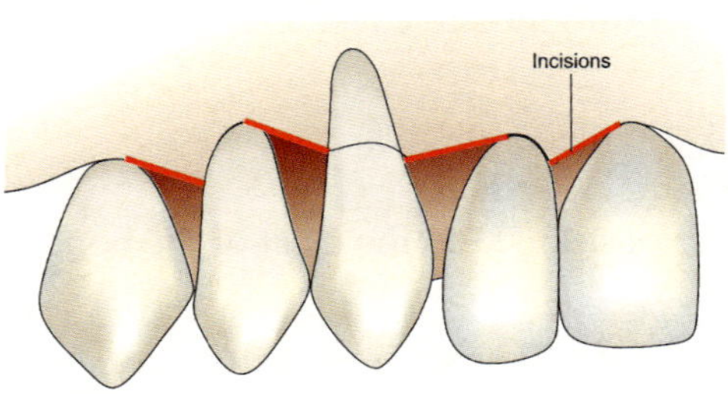

Fig. 11.3: Zuccheli technique: During coronal advancement, papilla mesial to the midline of the flap rotated in mesial coronal direction, papilla distal to midline rotated distal coronally

Free Gingival Graft to Increase the Width of Attached Gingiva (Figs 11.4a to f)

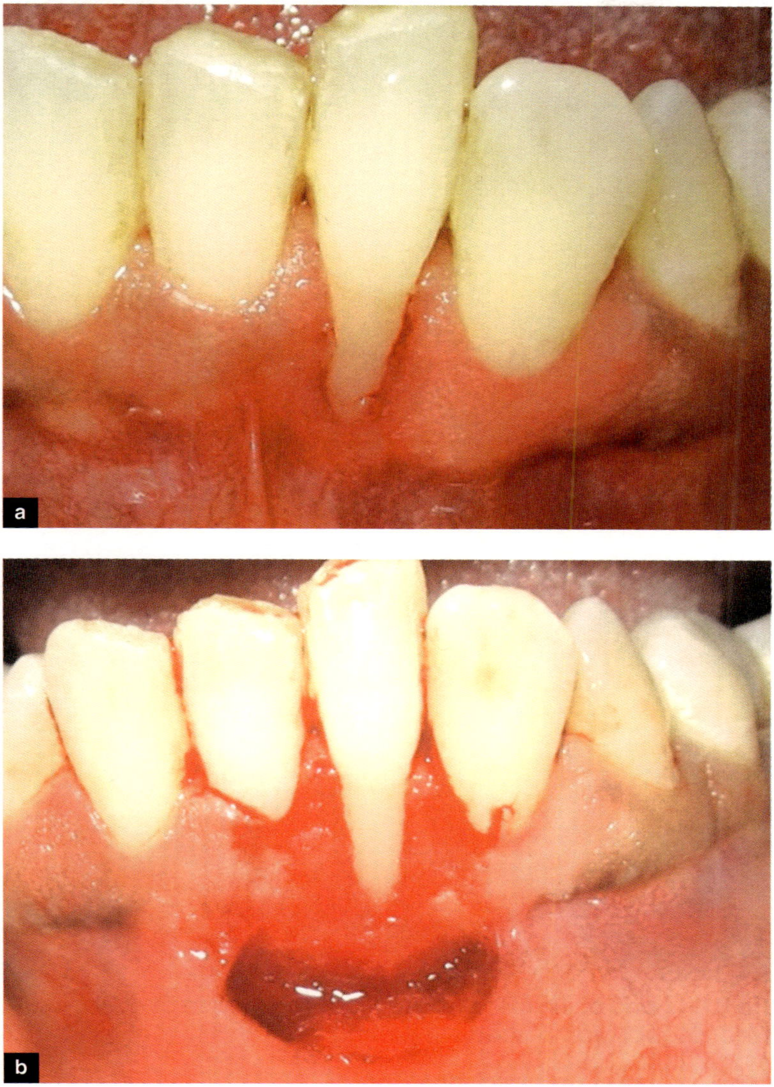

Fig. 11.4a and b: Miller class II recession-31. Recipient bed prepared—stab incision at MGJ

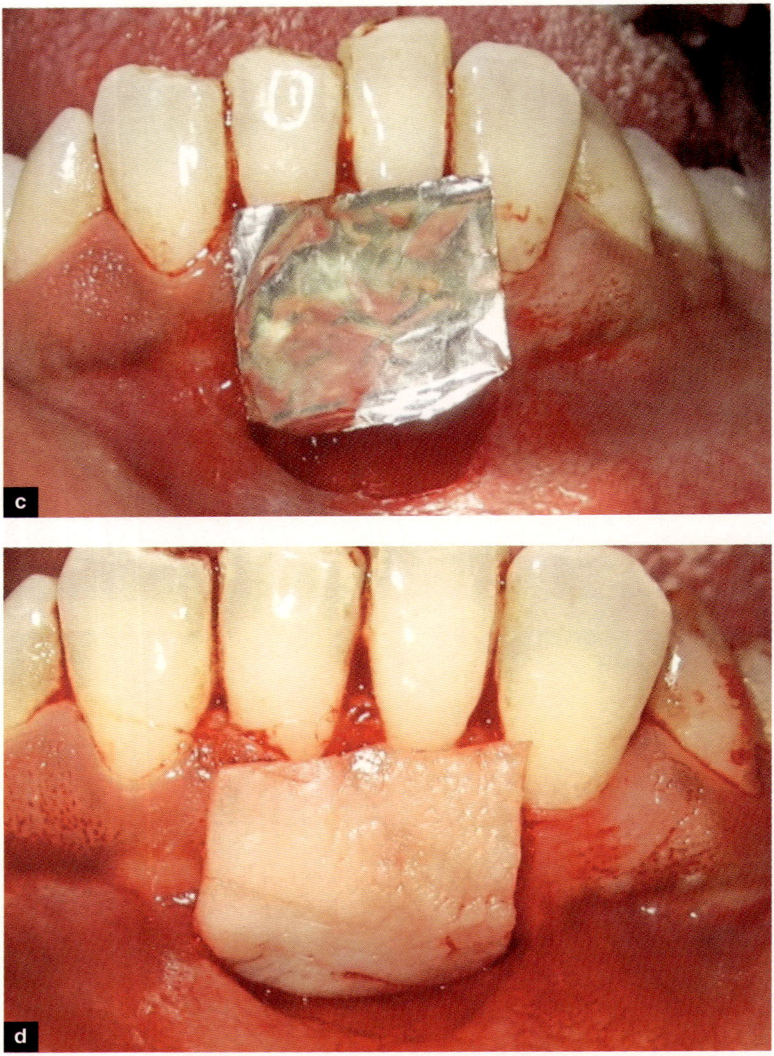

Fig. 11.4c and d: Tin foil template to outline the size of donor tissue. Free gingival graft placed

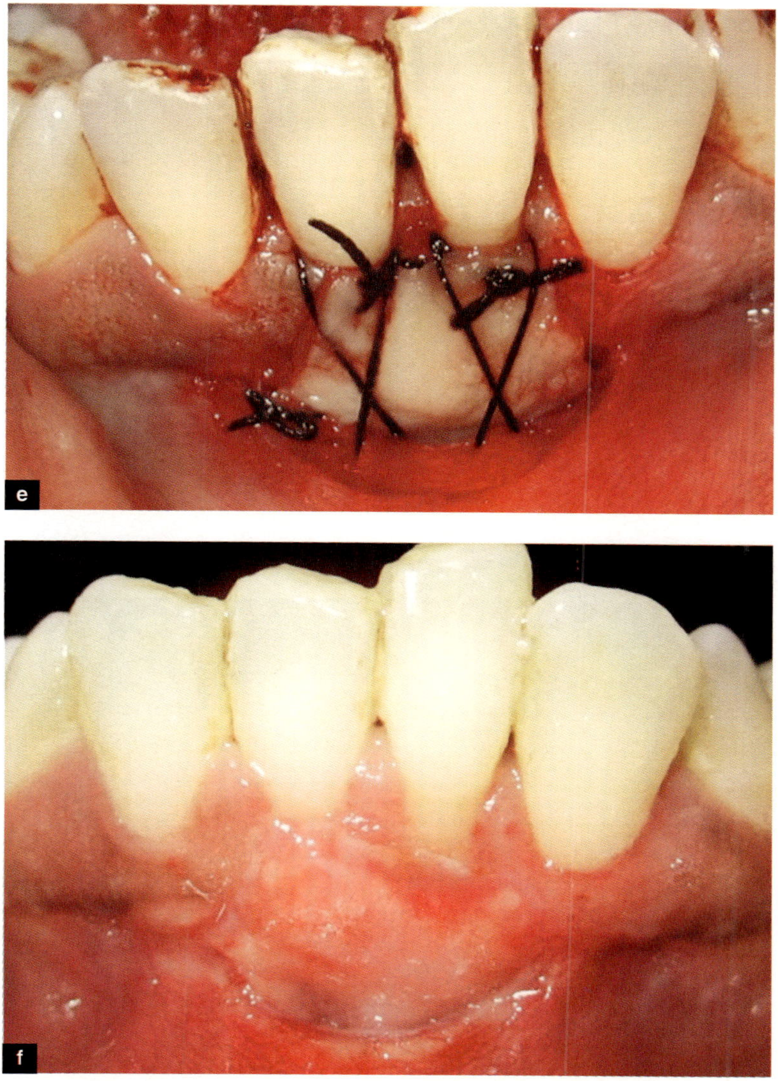

Fig. 11.4e and f: Circumferential sutures. Postoperative after 3 months

Connective Tissue Graft Accordion Technique (Fig. 11.5a to h)

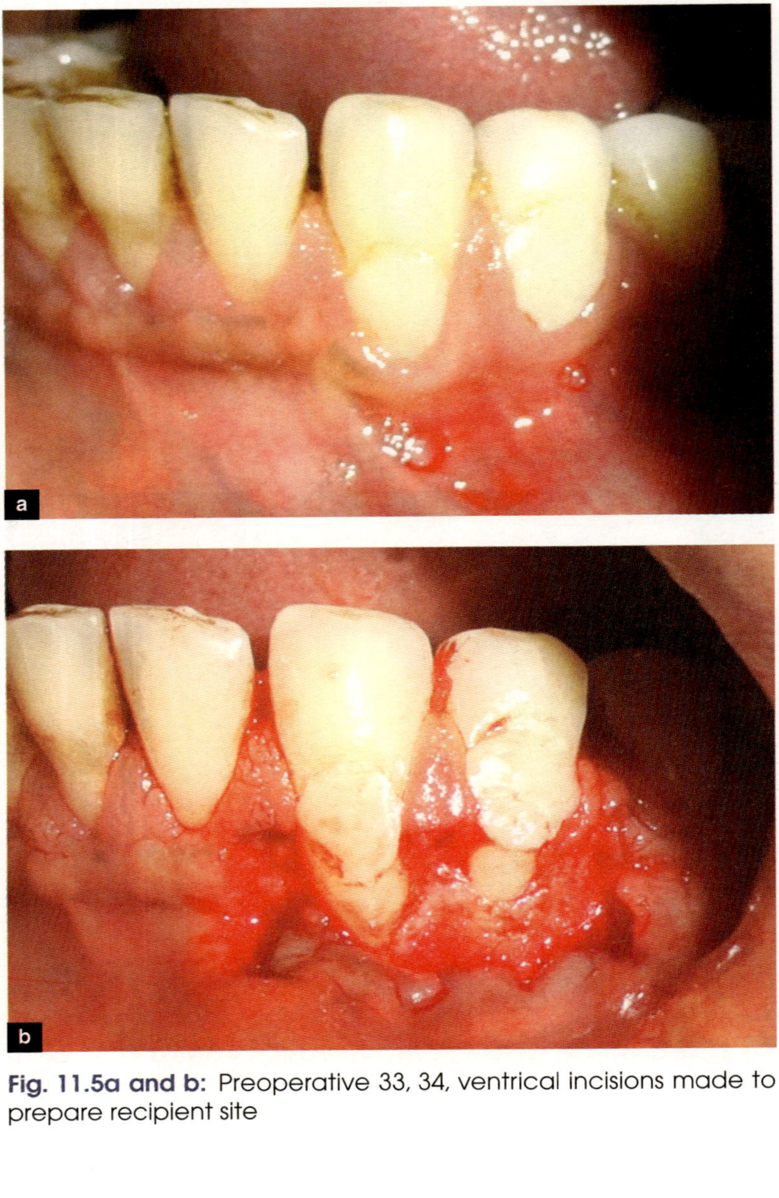

Fig. 11.5a and b: Preoperative 33, 34, ventrical incisions made to prepare recipient site

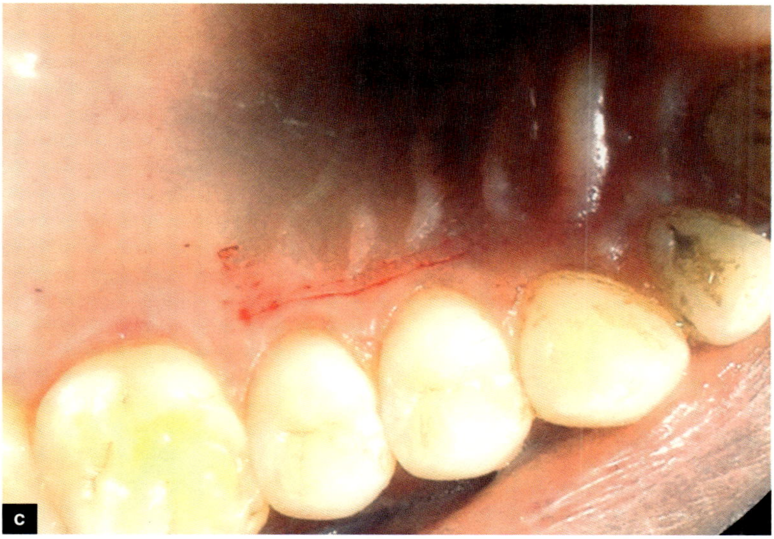

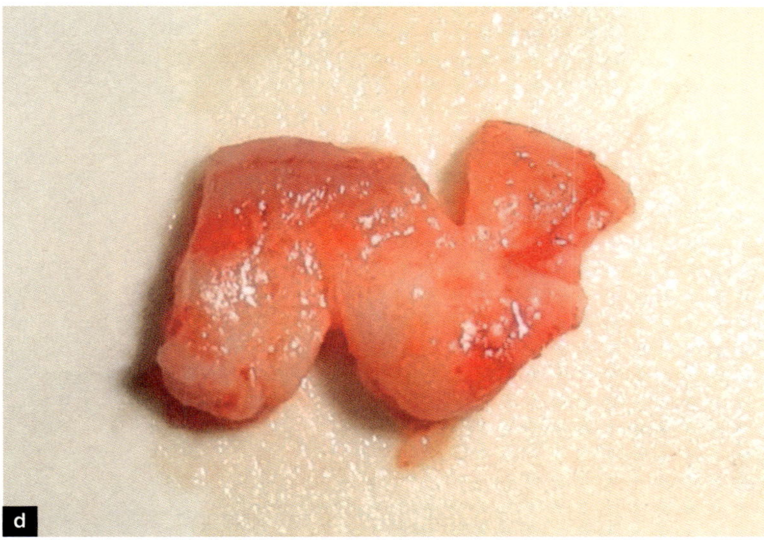

Fig. 11.5c and d: Connective tissue harvested in accordion technique

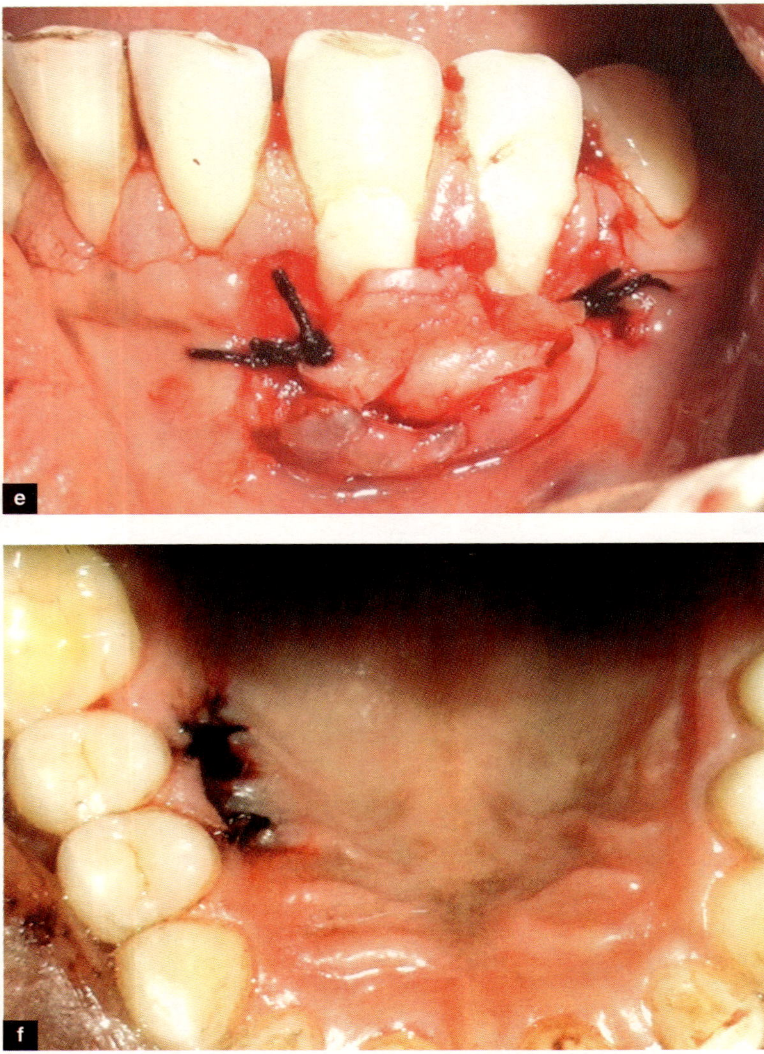

Fig. 11.5e and f: Suturing at the recipient site and palate done

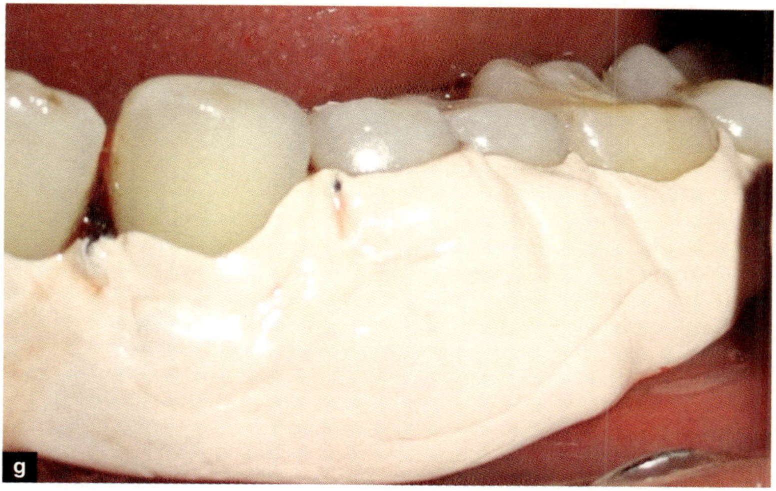

Fig. 11.5g: Coe pack placed

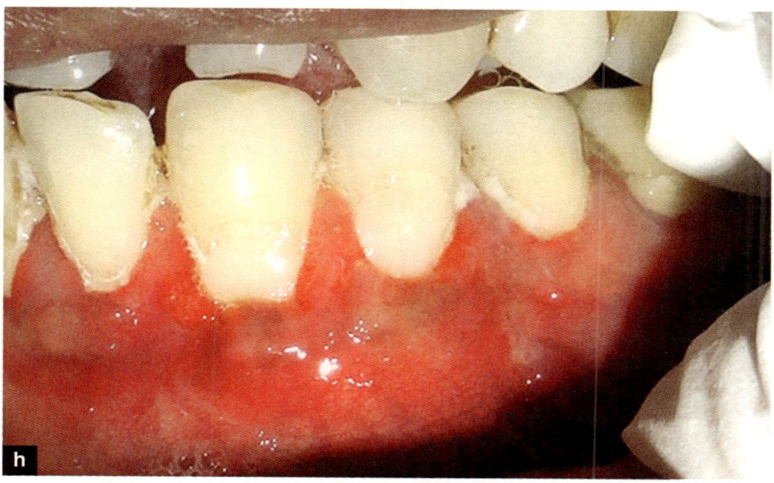

Fig. 11.5h: Postoperative after 1 month

Connective Tissue with Single Incision with Coronally Positioned Flap (Fig. 11.6a to h)

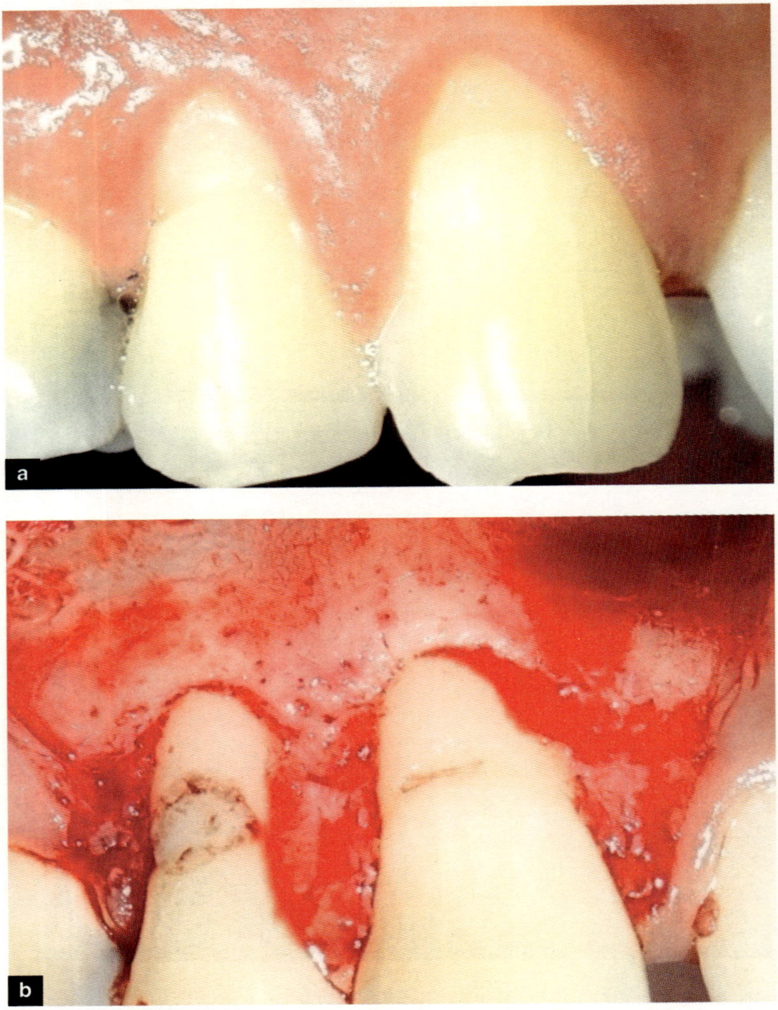

Fig. 11.6a and b: Preoperative 13, 14, vertical incisions made to raise a full thickness flap

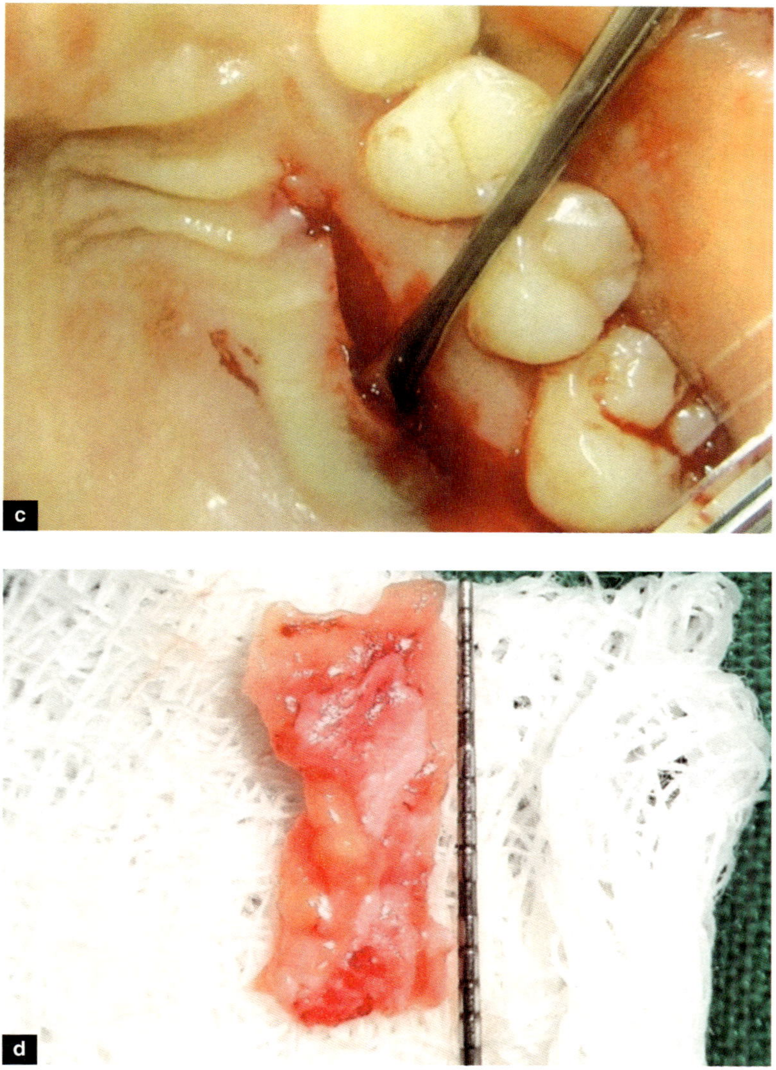

Fig. 11.6c and d: Connective tissue harvested from palate

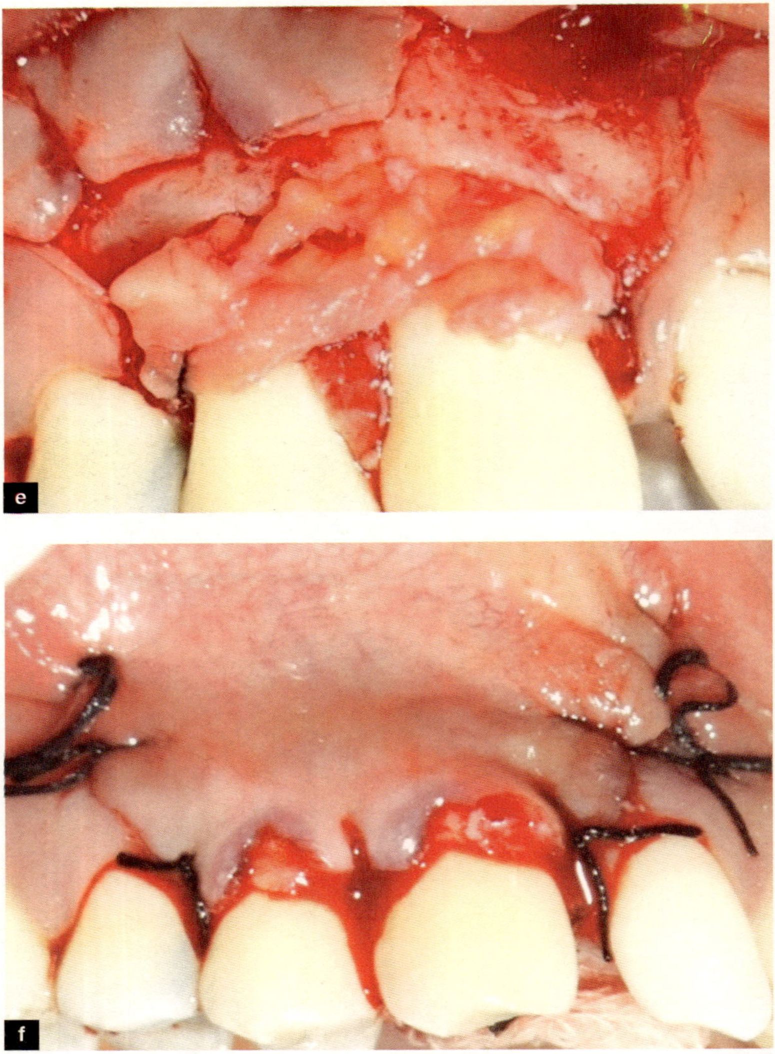

Fig. 11.6e and f: Connective tissue placed at the recipient site and sutured

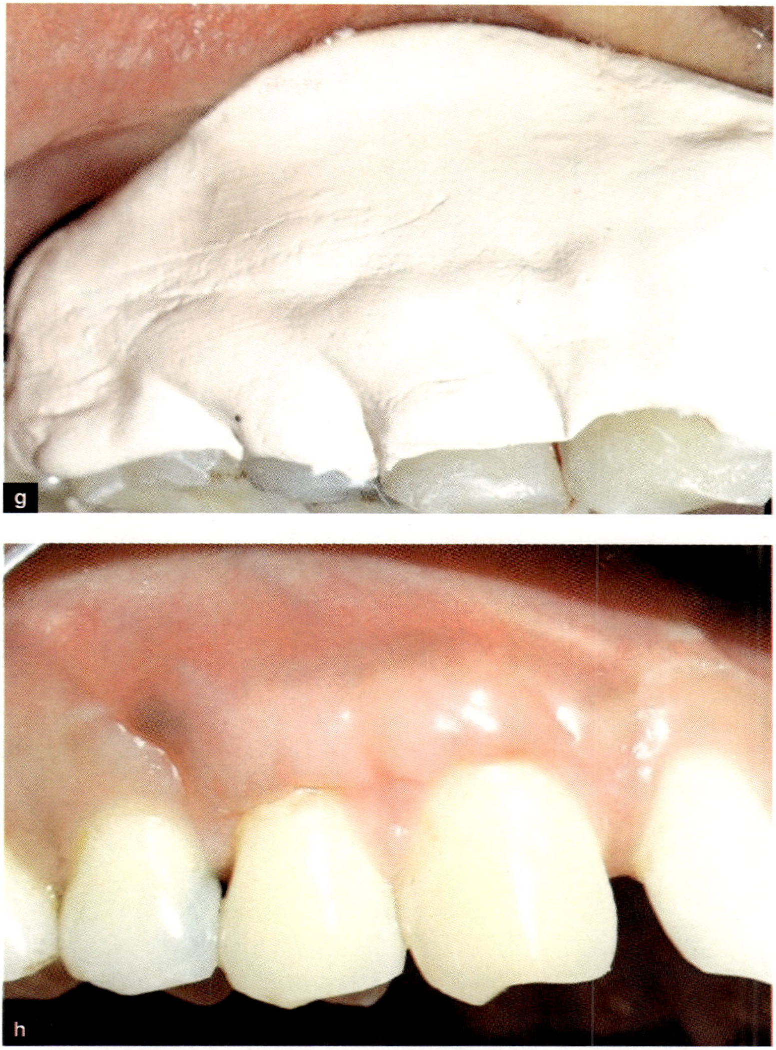

Fig. 11.6g and h: Coe pack placed. Postoperative after 1 month

Connective Tissue with Pouch (Fig. 11.7a to f)

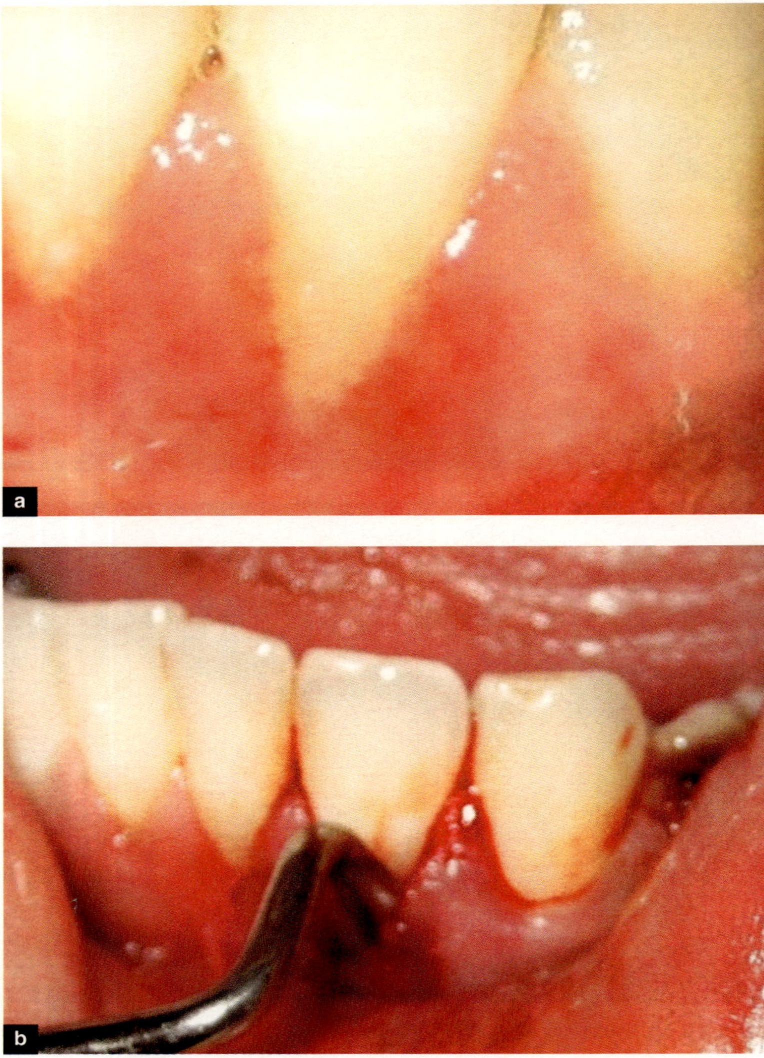

Fig. 11.7a and b: Miller's class I recession 33. Pouch preparation done. Space created with Orban's knife

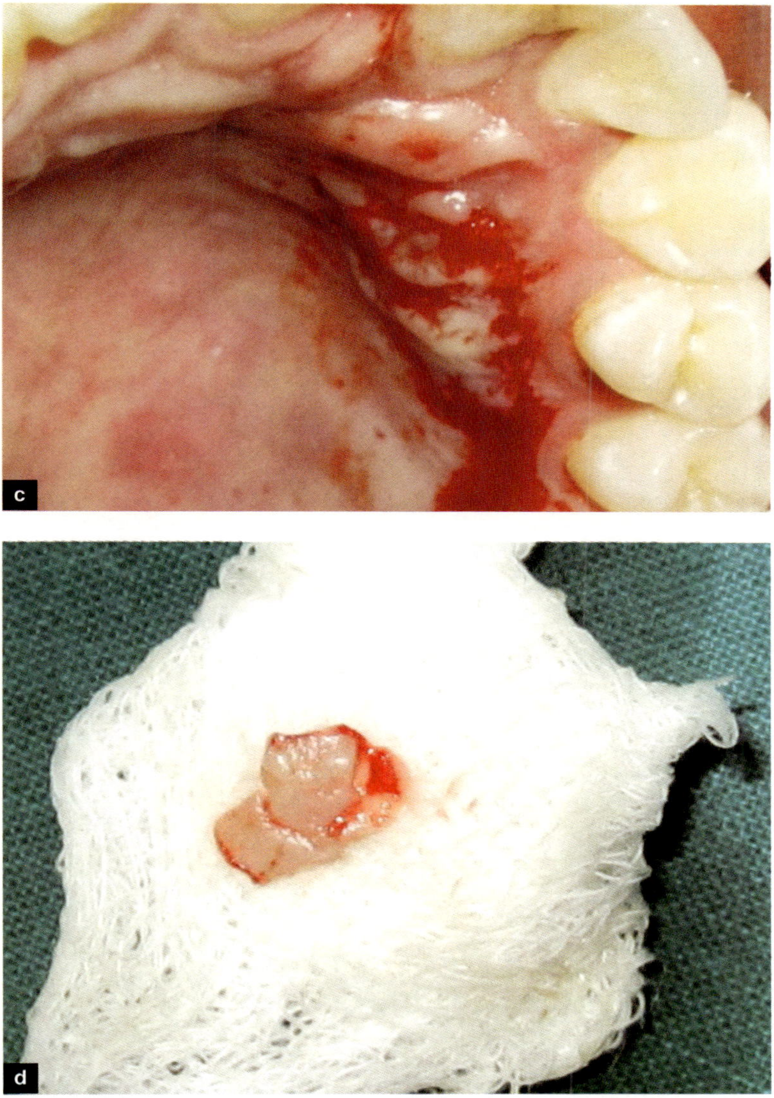

Fig. 11.7c and d: Incisions for Trap door technique of harvesting CT

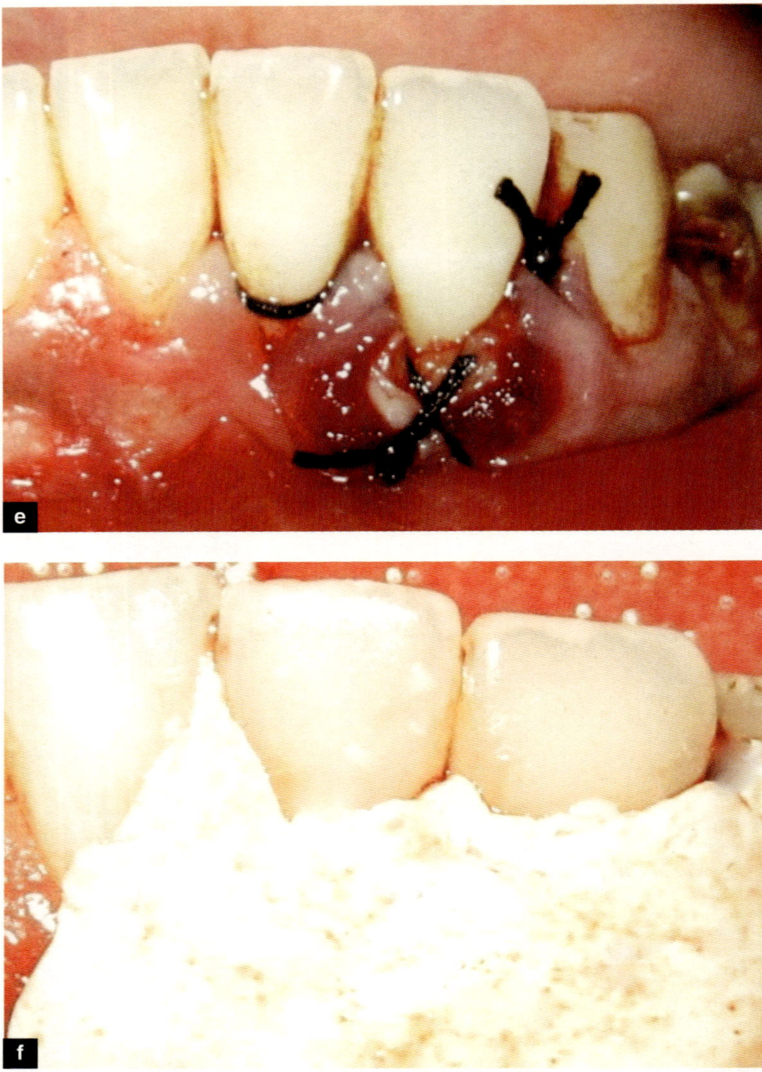

Fig. 11.7e and f: Suturing done and periodontal pack placed

Semilunar Advanced Flap (Fig. 11.8a to f)

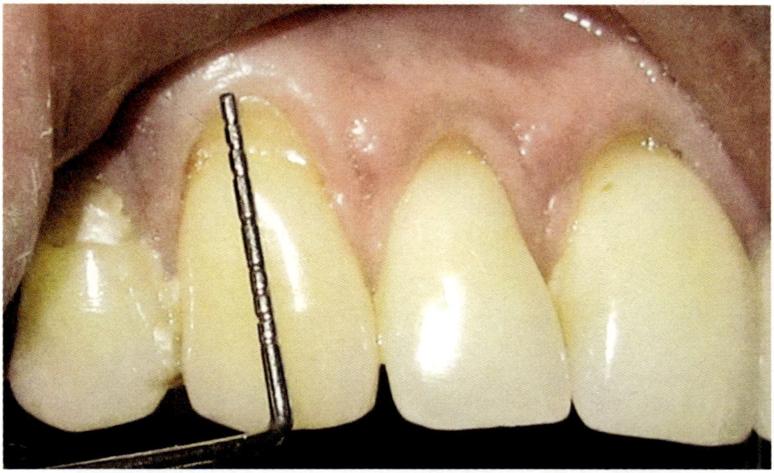

Fig. 11.8a: Miller's recession class I 13—height 3 mm

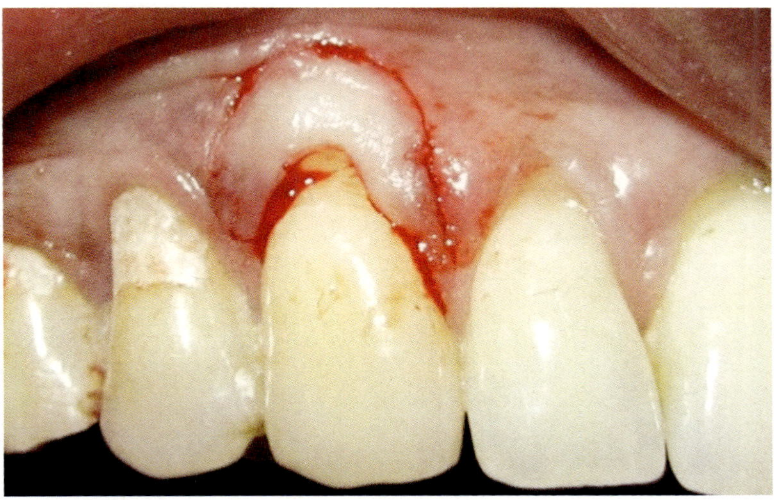

Fig. 11.8b: Semilunar incision placed. Partial thickness flap raised

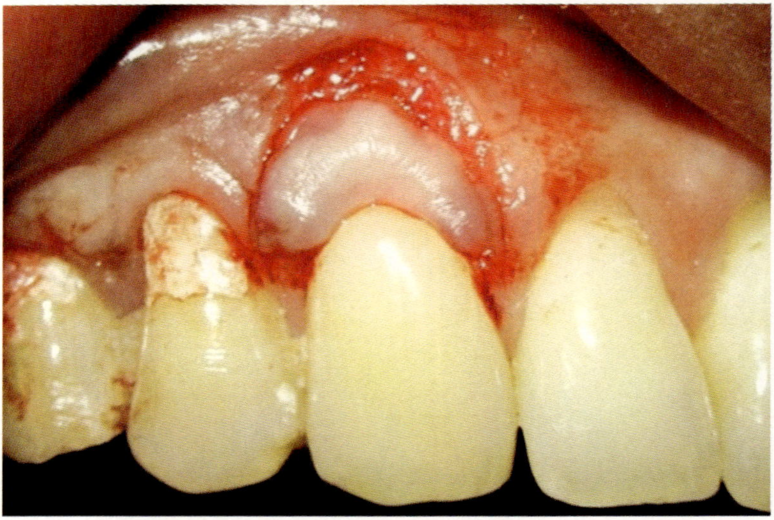

Fig. 11.8c: Coronal advancement of the flap done

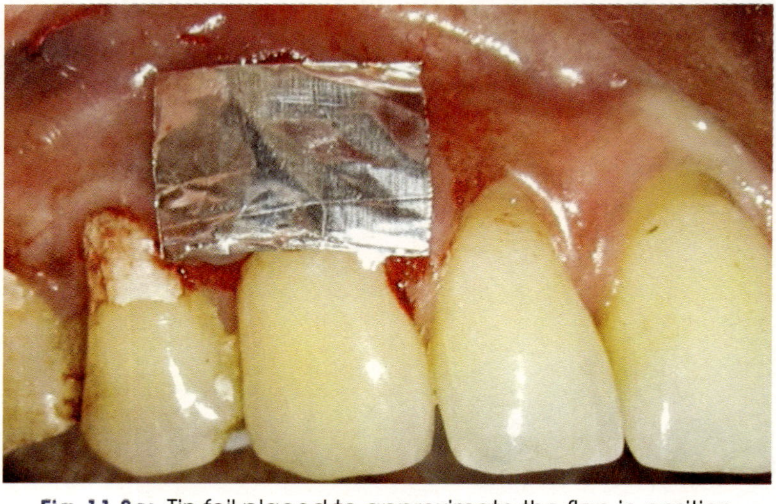

Fig. 11.8c: Tin foil placed to approximate the flap in position

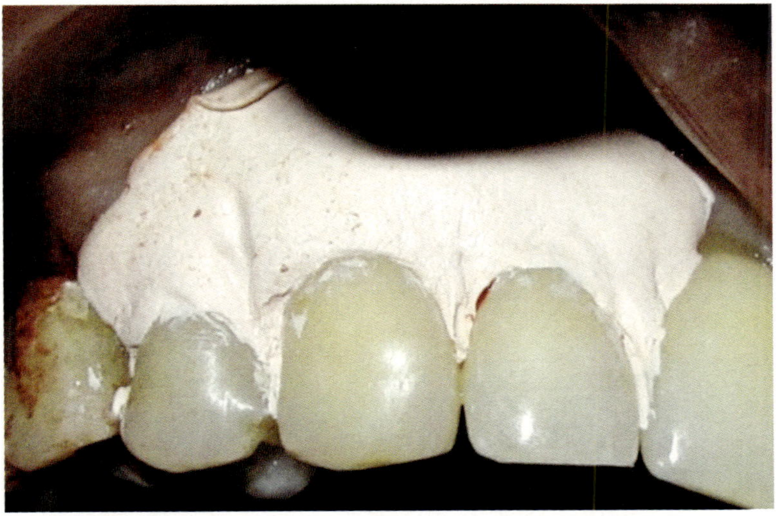

Fig. 11.8e: Periodontal pack placement done

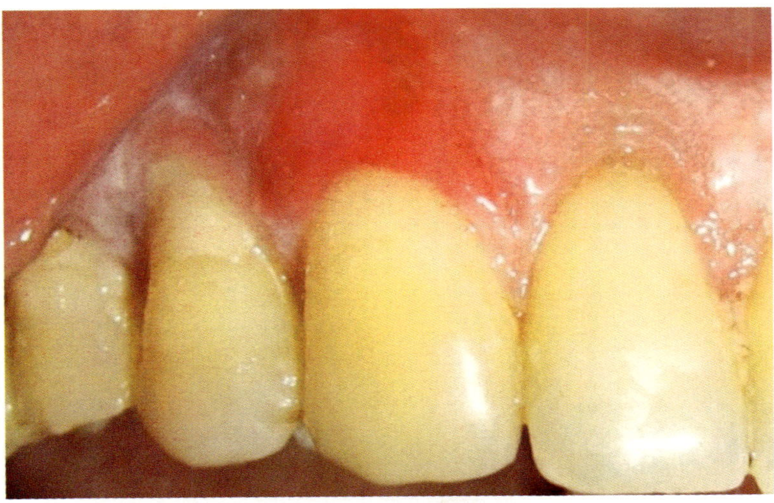

Fig. 11.8f: Postoperative after 1 month

Coronally Advanced Flap (Fig. 11.9a to f)

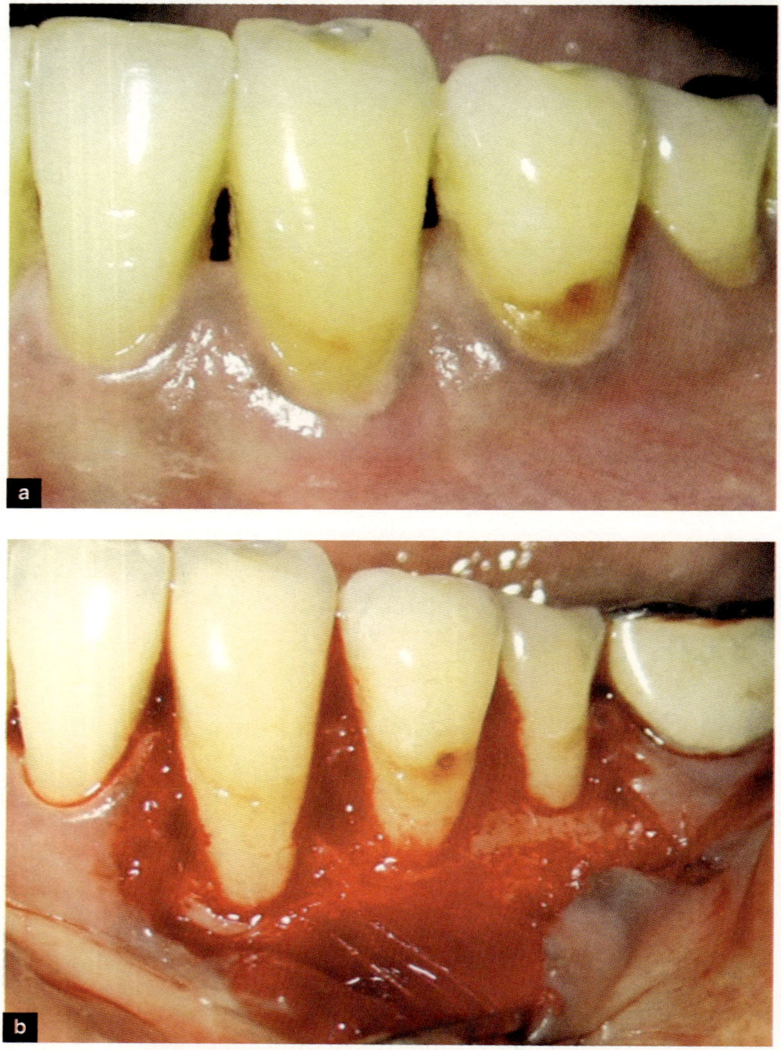

Fig. 11.9a and b: Miller's class I recession-14, 15. Full thickness flap raised with marginal and vertical incisions

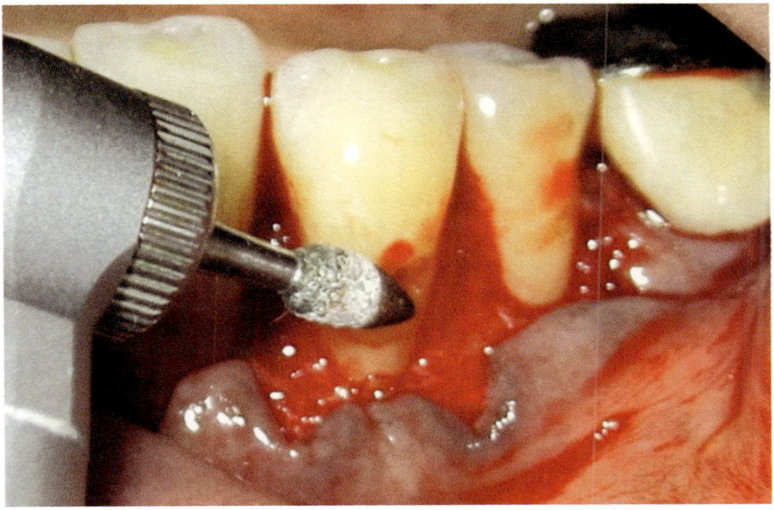

Fig. 11.9c: Odontoplasty done to smoothen the root prominence

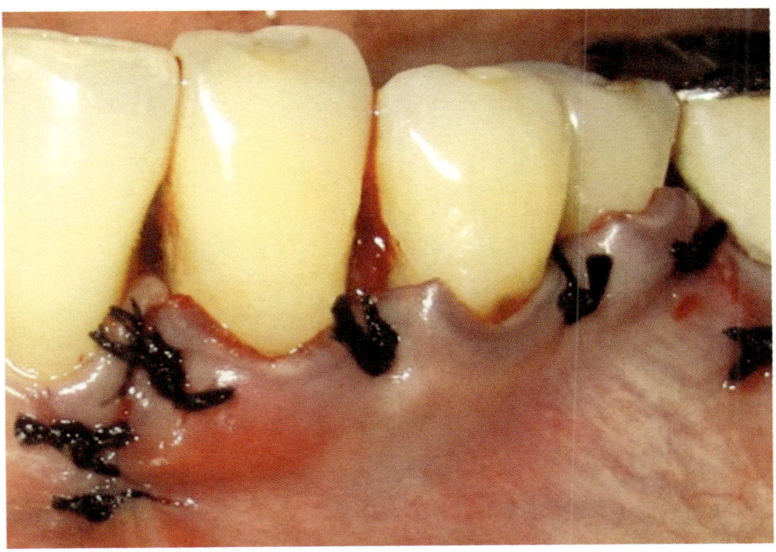

Fig. 11.9d: Flap colonially positioned and sutured

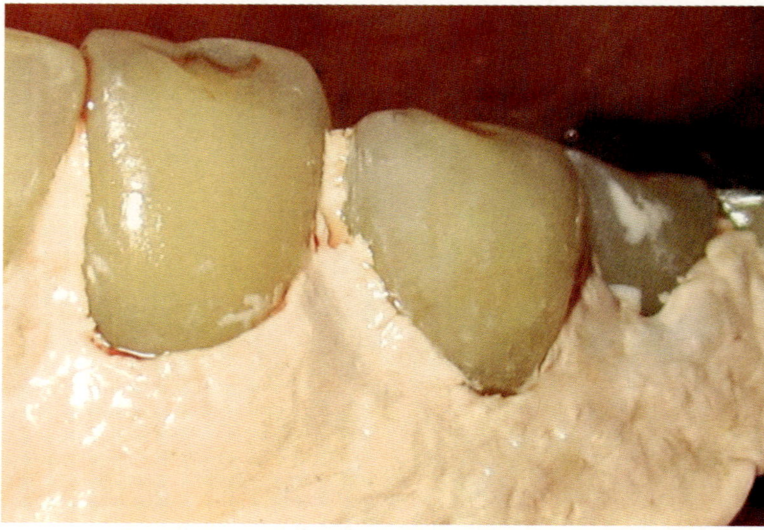

Fig. 11.9e: Coe pack placed

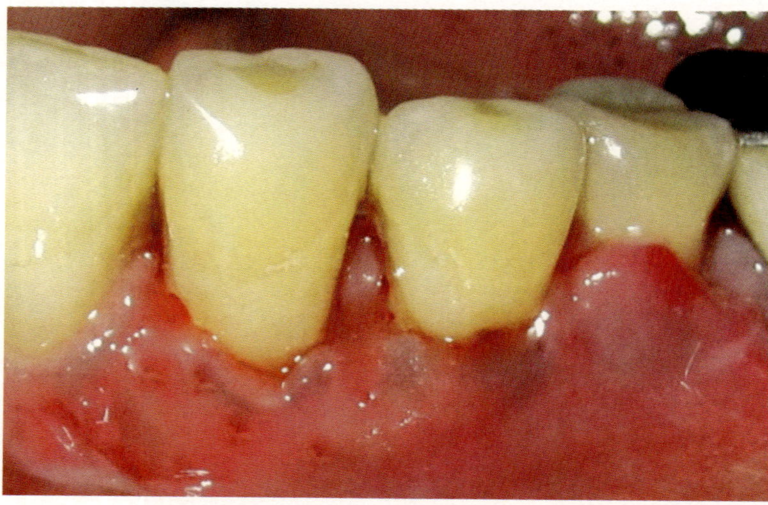

Fig. 11.9f: Postoperative after 1 month

Modified Coronally Positioned Flap for Multiple Recessions (Fig. 11.10a to f)

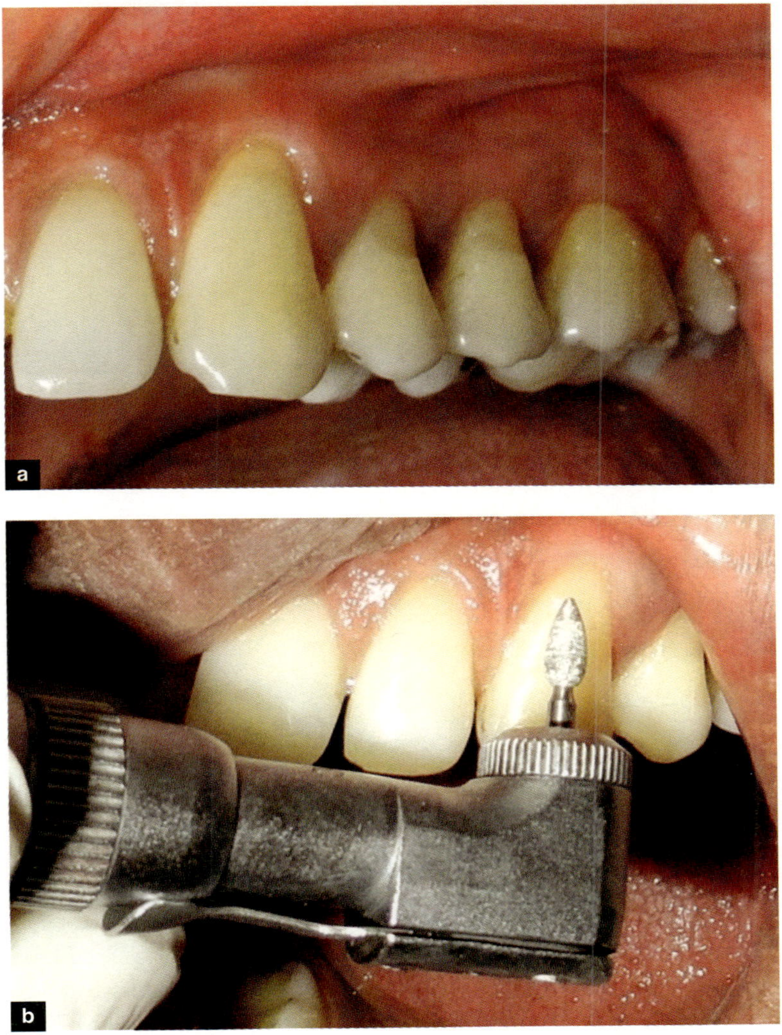

Fig. 11.10a and b: Miller's class I recession 13, 14, 15. Osteoplasty done to remove root prominence

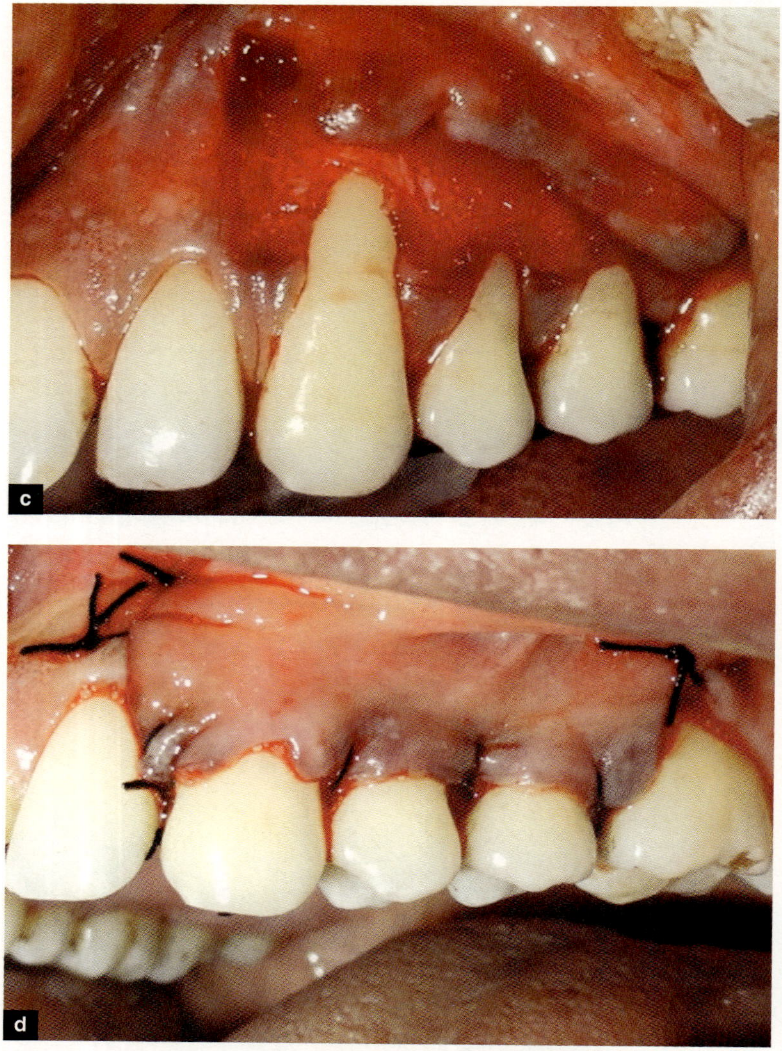

Fig. 11.10c and d: Submarginal and vertical incisions to raise modified coronally positioned flap. Single interrupted suturing done

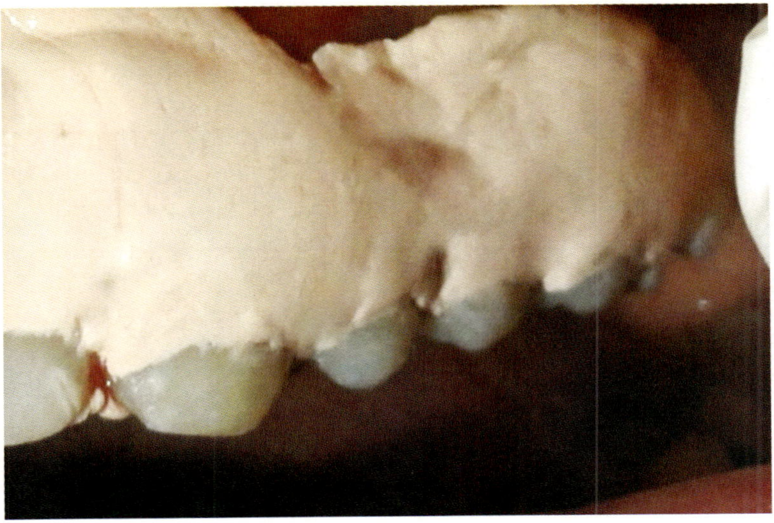

Fig. 11.10e: Coe pack placed

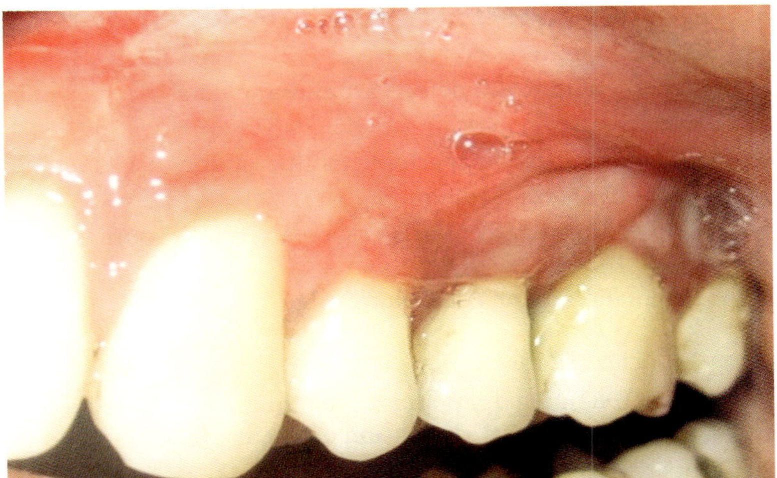

Fig. 11.10f: Postoperative root coverage after 1 year

12

Periodontal Plastic Surgery

DEFINITION

Surgical procedures performed to prevent or correct anatomical, developmental, traumatic or plaque induced defects of the gingiva, alveolar mucosa or bone (proceedings of world workshop in periodontics, 1996).

Periodontal Plastic Surgery Procedures

a. Gingival augmentation
b. Root coverage/recession coverage
c. Correction of mucosal defects around implants
d. Crown lengthening
e. Gingival preservation at ectopic tooth eruption
f. Removal of aberrant frenum
g. Prevention of ridge collapse associated with tooth extraction
h. Augmentation of the edentulous ridge

I. Inadequate Gingival Width

Friedman (1962); De Trey and Bernimoulin (1980): Adequate amount of gingiva is any dimension of gingiva that is:

1. Compatible with gingival health, or
2. Prevents retraction of the gingival margin during movements of the alveolar mucosa.

Note: *Commonly agreed that areas with less than 2 mm of attached gingiva are at a higher risk for recession* ***(Lindhe and Nyman, 1980).***

Clinical Note

Tissue barrier concept by Goldman and Cohen (1979): They recommended that dense band of connective tissue serves as a thick barrier against spread of inflammation. Hence, an adequate tissue barrier should be maintained by increasing the zone of keratinized gingiva (attached gingiva).

Tension test—to establish whether the gingival and oral mucosa complex is adequate for the maintenance of gingival health.

Clinical Note

1. *It is important to remember that any dimension of gingiva can be maintained healthy by the patient.*
2. *Surgical procedures to treat inadequate (<1 mm) of attached gingiva is only indicated if:*
   - *There is an active site of recession,*
   - *Patient experiences discomfort during toothbrushing and/or chewing due to interfering lining mucosa,*
   - *Patient is undergoing restorative/orthodontic procedures*

Treatment modalities for correction of inadequate gingiva

a. Denudation technique
b. Periosteal retention
c. Vestibular extension procedure
d. Apically displaced flap
e. Free gingival grafts

II. High Frenum and its Correction

Depending upon the attachment level, frenum has been classified as: (Placek et al., 1974)

- Mucosal
- Gingival
- Papillary
- Papillary penetrating

Frenectomy is a complete removal of the frenum, including its attachment to the underlying bone (Fig. 12.1), and may be required for correction of abnormal diastema between maxillary central incisors (Friedman, 1957).

Frenotomy is the incision and relocation of the frenal attachment.

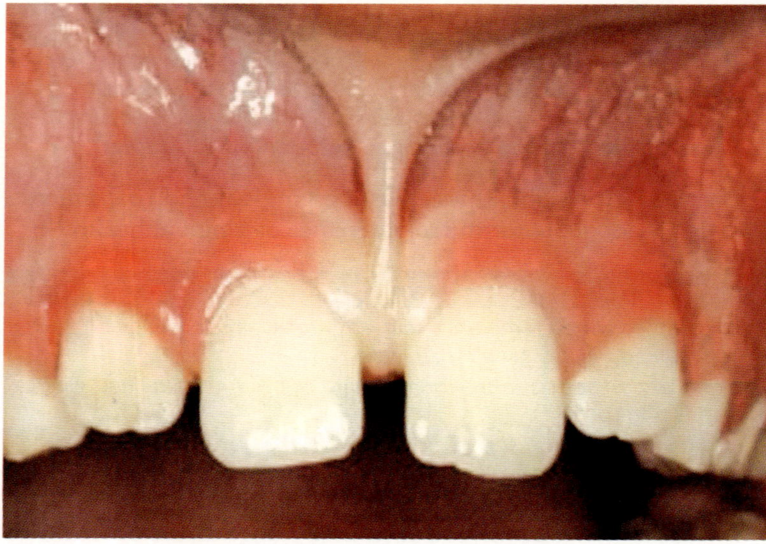

Fig. 12.1: High frenal attachment between maxillary central incisors

Conventional frenectomy technique.
- Dieffenbach—V plasty
- Schuchardt and Mathis—Z plasty

III. Gummy Smile

Garber and Salama (1996) classification for excessive gingival display and their proposed treatments.

a. *Degree I:* 2 to 4 mm of gingival display. Treatment would be orthodontic intrusion alone, orthodontics and crown lengthening or crown lengthening followed by restorations.
b. *Degree II:* 4 to 8 mm of gingival display. Treatment would be crown lengthening and restorations or orthognathic surgery depending on the crown/root ratio.
c. *Degree III:* >8 mm of gingival display. Treatment would be orthognathic surgery with or without crown lengthening and restorative treatment.

IV. Altered Passive Eruption

Active eruption: It is the occlusal movement of a tooth as it emerges from its crypt in the gingiva.

Clinical Note (Lindhe, 3rd ed)

1. *In young patients with adequate width of attached gingiva and >1 mm of free gingiva, complaint of small front teeth and a thin periodontal biotype, full exposure of the anatomic crown can be accomplished by a gingivectomy/gingivoplasty procedure.*
2. *To solve aesthetic problems in patients who have short anatomic crowns in the anterior section of the dentition, extensive bone recontouring is required.*

2a. ***Subjects who have normal occlusal relationships****—the clinical crowns can be made longer by surgically exposing root structure and by locating the cervical margins of the restorations apical to the CEJ.*

2b. ***Subjects who have abnormal occlusal relationships with excessive*** *interocclusal space in the posterior dentition when the anterior teeth are in* **edge-to-edge contact***—the length of the maxillary front teeth can be reduced. The marginal gingiva can be resected or relocated to an apical position before crown restorations are made.*

Passive eruption: It is characterized by the apical shift of the dentogingival junction. As this occurs, the length of the clinical crown increases, with the apical migration of the epithelial attachment **(Gottlieb and Orban, 1933) (Fig. 12.2).**

Altered passive eruption (APE) is a clinical situation produced by excessive gum overlapping over the enamel limits, resulting in a short clinical crown appearance that gives the sensation of hidden teeth.

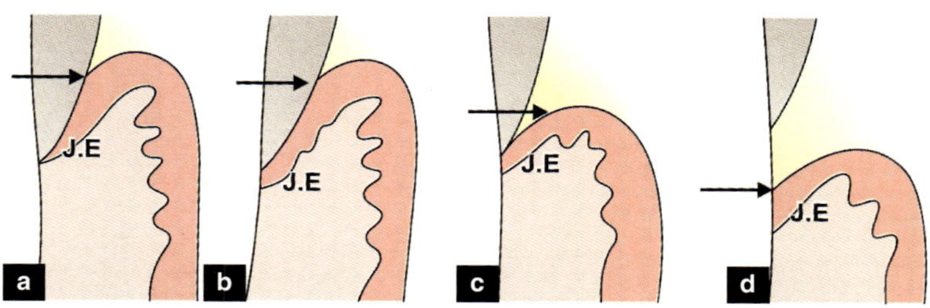

Fig. 12.2a to d: Four steps in passive eruption. (a) Base of gingival sulcus and JE are on enamel; (b) Base of gingiva sulcus is on enamel and JE is on root; (c) Base of sulcus is at cement enamel line and entire JE is on root; (d) Base of gingival sulcus and JE are on root

Altered passive eruption has been classified by *Coslet et al*, 1977 (Fig. 12.3) as:

Based on gingival–anatomic crown relationship:

a. *Type I:* Gingival margin is incisal/occlusal to CEJ. **There is a noticeable wider gingival dimension** from the margin to mucogingival junction.
b. *Type II:* **Dimension** from the gingival margin to the mucogingival junction **appears to be within the normal mean** width.

Based on alveolar crest CEJ relationship, Type 1 and Type II are further subdivided as:

a. *Subtype A:* The alveolar crest—CEJ distance is approximately 1.5 mm. This allows for normal attachment of gingival fibers into cementum.
b. *Subtype B:* The alveolar crest is at the level of the CEJ.

Clinical Note

Clinically a patient with altered passive eruption presents with a gummy smile and short clinical crowns. However, features like short/ hyperactive maxillary lip, dentoalveolar extrusion, vertical maxillary excess or a combination of these can help in confirmation of passive eruption.

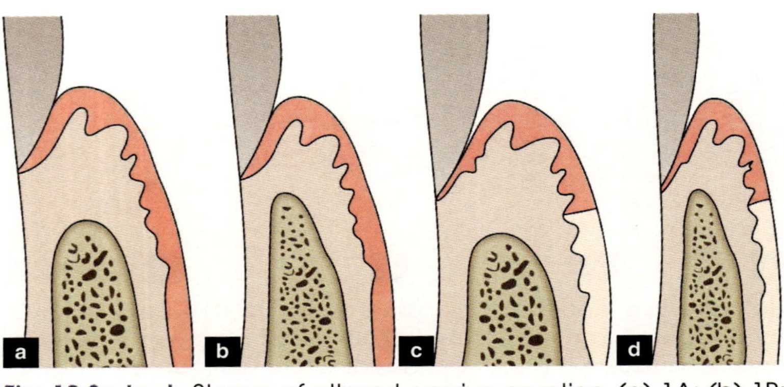

Fig. 12.3a to d: Stages of altered passive eruption. (a) 1A; (b) 1B; (c) 2A; (d) 2B

V. Surgical Exposure of Impacted Teeth

a. Maxillary and mandibular third molars are the most commonly impacted teeth due to their long development time.
b. The maxillary cuspid is the second most frequently impacted tooth (2%).

   Four criteria to determine method for uncovering the tooth:

   a. Ist criterion—assess the labiolingual position of impacted crown
   b. IInd criterion—evaluate is the vertical position of the tooth relative to the mucogingival junction.
   c. IIIrd criterion—evaluate the amount of gingiva in the area of the impacted canine.
   d. IV criterion—evaluate the mesiodistal position of the canine crown

   Most commonly used technique for uncovering of impacted teeth is open eruption (window technique).

Clinical Note for Technique (Lindhe, 3rd ed)

1. *Double pedicle graft:* This flap procedure is indicated when the permanent tooth erupts within the zone of keratinized tissue but close to the mucogingival junction.
2. *Apically positioned flap:* When the permanent tooth is erupting apical to the mucogingival junction, vertical releasing incisions have to be placed to allow for apical positioning of the keratinized tissue.
3. *Free gingival graft:* If the tooth is erupting within the alveolar mucosa distant to the mucogingival junction, a free gingival graft procedure may be selected. The entrapped gingiva is removed by a split incision and used as an epithelialized connective tissue graft.

VI. Interdental Papilla Reconstruction (Fig. 12.4)

Nordland and Tarnow (1998) proposed a classification system regarding the papillary height adjacent to natural teeth, based on three anatomic landmarks: Interdental contact point, apical extent of the facial CEJ, and coronal extent of the proximal CEJ.

1. *Normal:* The interdental papilla occupies the entire embrasure space apical to the interdental contact point/area.
2. *Class I:* The tip of the interdental papilla is located between the interdental contact point and the level of the CEJ on the proximal surface of the tooth.

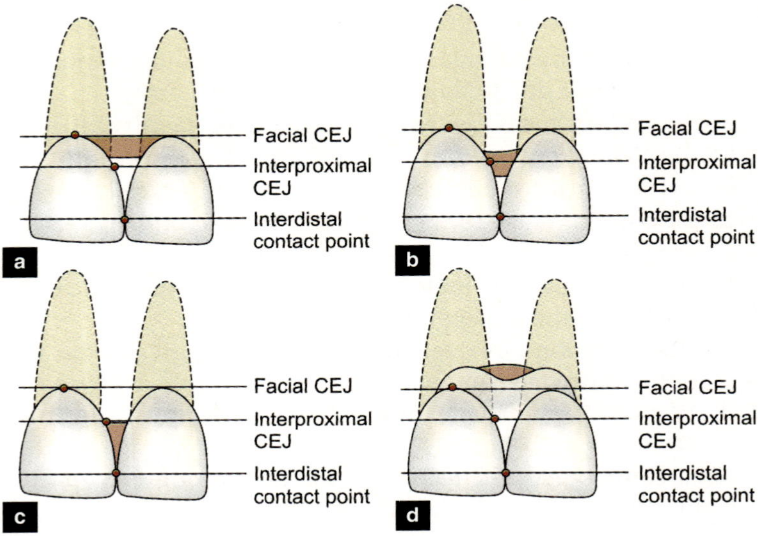

Fig. 12.4a to d: Classification system for papilla height. (a) Normal; (b) Class I; (c) Class II; (d) Class III

3. *Class II:* The tip of the interdental papilla is located at or apical to the level of the CEJ on the proximal surface of the tooth but coronal to the level of the CEJ mid-buccally.
4. *Class III:* The tip of the interdental papilla is located at or apical to the level of the CEJ mid-buccally.

Clinical Note for Postgraduates

1. *To surgically reconstruct an interdental papilla, following two points should be kept in mind (Lindhe, 3rd ed)*
    a. *The vertical distance between the bone crest and the apical point of the contact area between the crowns, and*
    b. *The soft tissue height in the interdental area.*

Surgical intervention: If the distance bone crestcontact point is ≤ 5 mm and the papilla height is less than 4 mm, surgery would be indicated for increasing the volume of the papilla and for the treatment of black triangle.

Lengthening the contact area apically: It is indicated If the contact point is located >5 mm from the bone crest, because of loss of periodontal support and/or an inappropriate interdental contact relationship between the crowns.

Eliminate/minimize traumatic injury to the papillae: If loss of papilla height is only caused by soft tissue damage from oral hygiene devices.

Lingual Frenectomy (Fig. 12.5a to f)

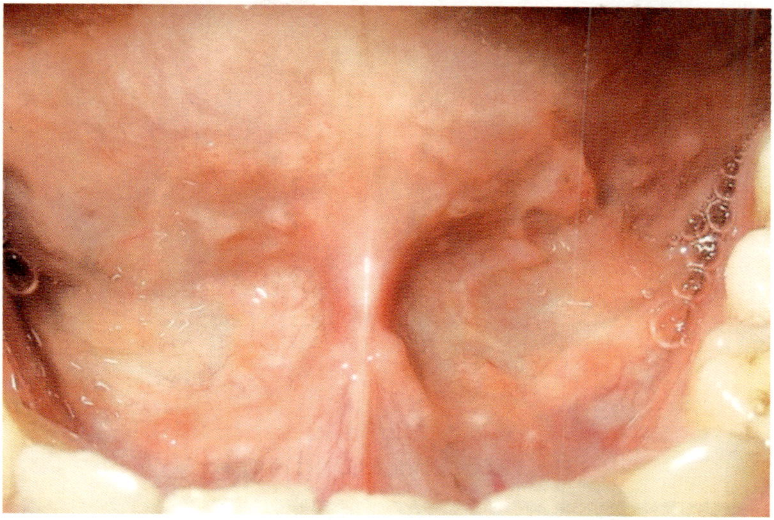

Fig. 12.5a: High lingual frenal attachment

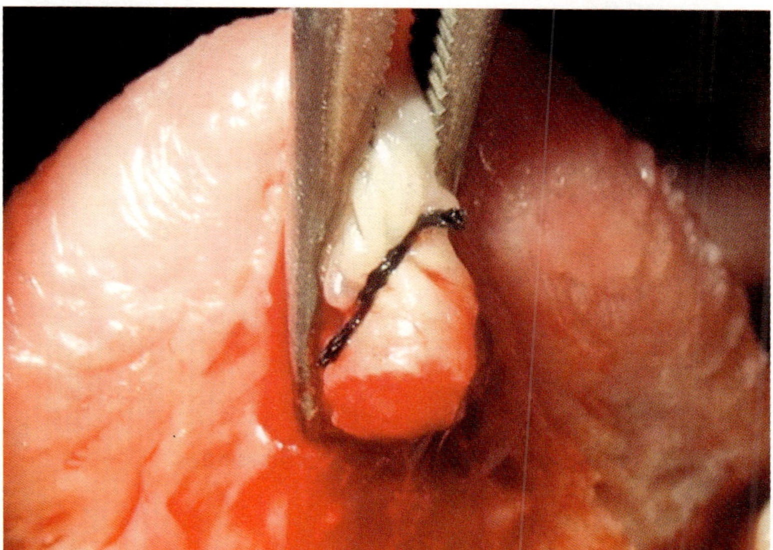

Fig. 12.5b: Presuturing and frenotomy

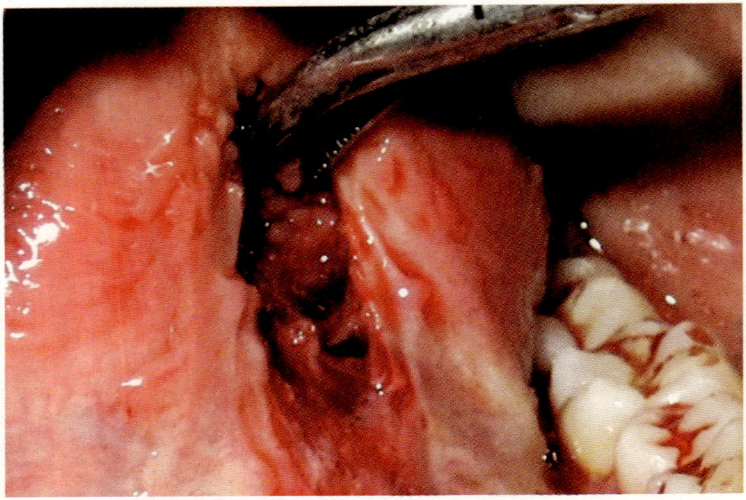

Fig. 12.5c: Undermining of fibers

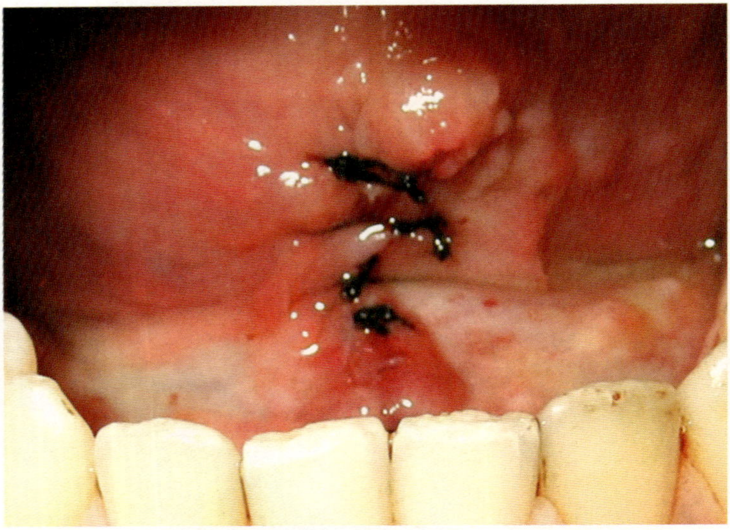

Fig. 12.5d: Single interrupted sutures

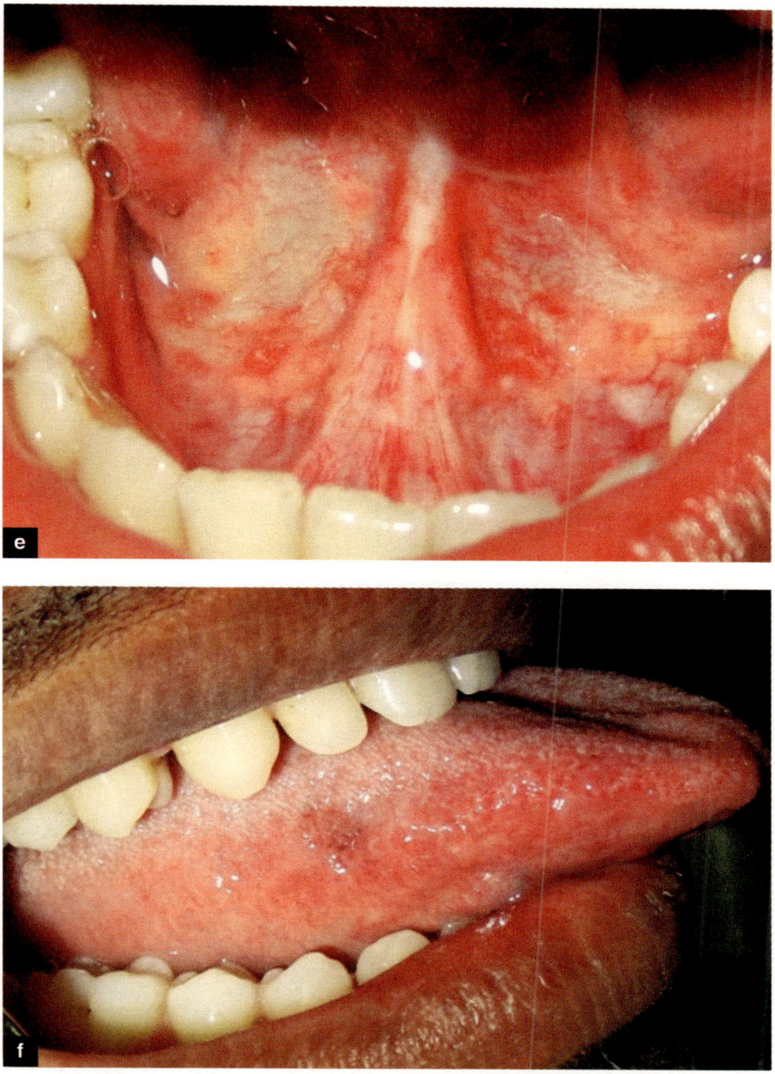

Fig. 12.5e and f: Postoperative after 15 days and increased tongue protrusion

Aesthetic Crown Lengthening (Fig. 12.6a to f)

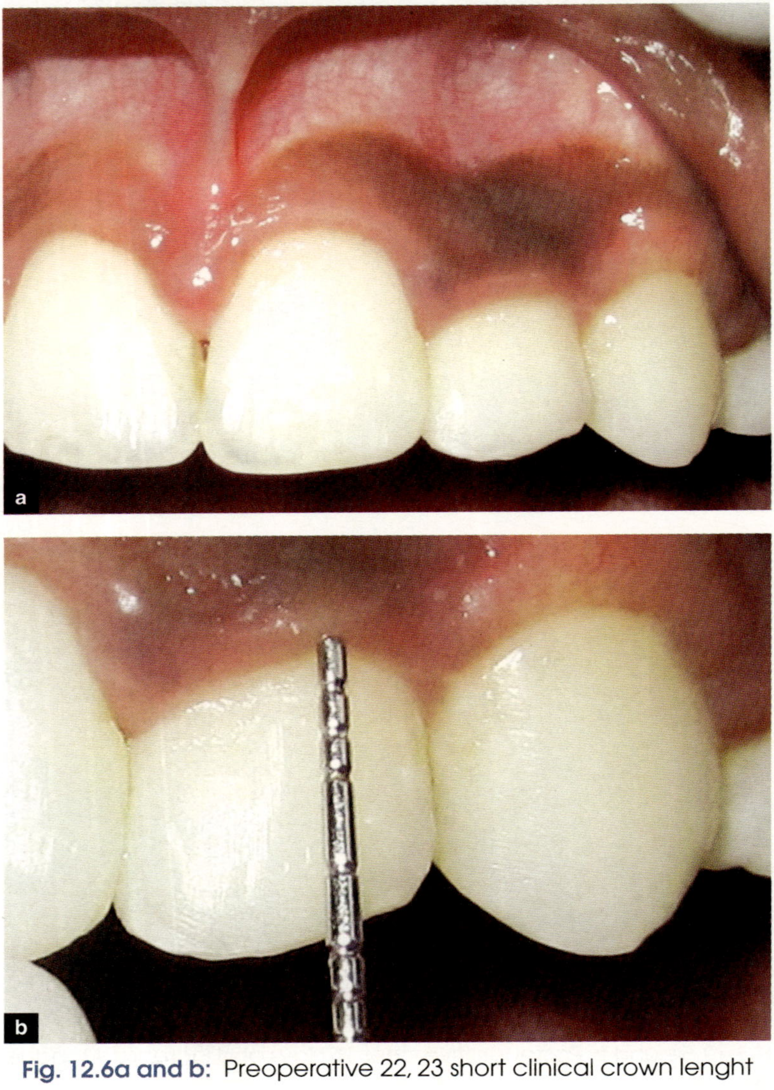

Fig. 12.6a and b: Preoperative 22, 23 short clinical crown lenght

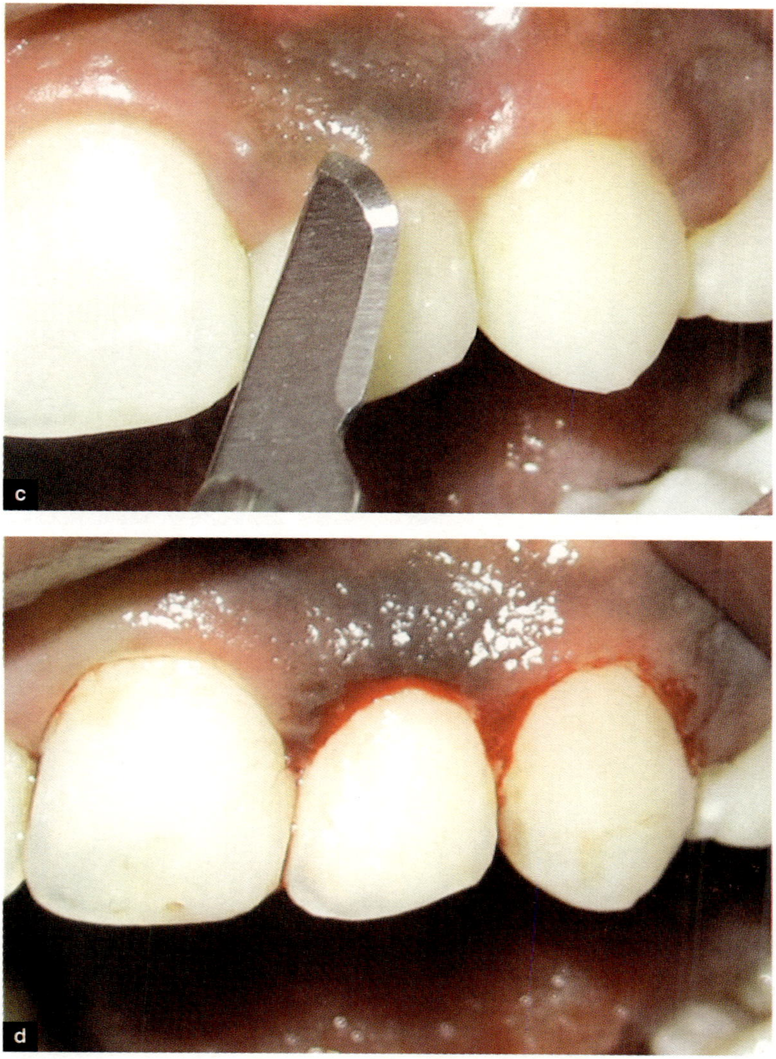

Fig. 12.6c and d: After bone sounding, excision of 2 m of gingival margin to expose the crown

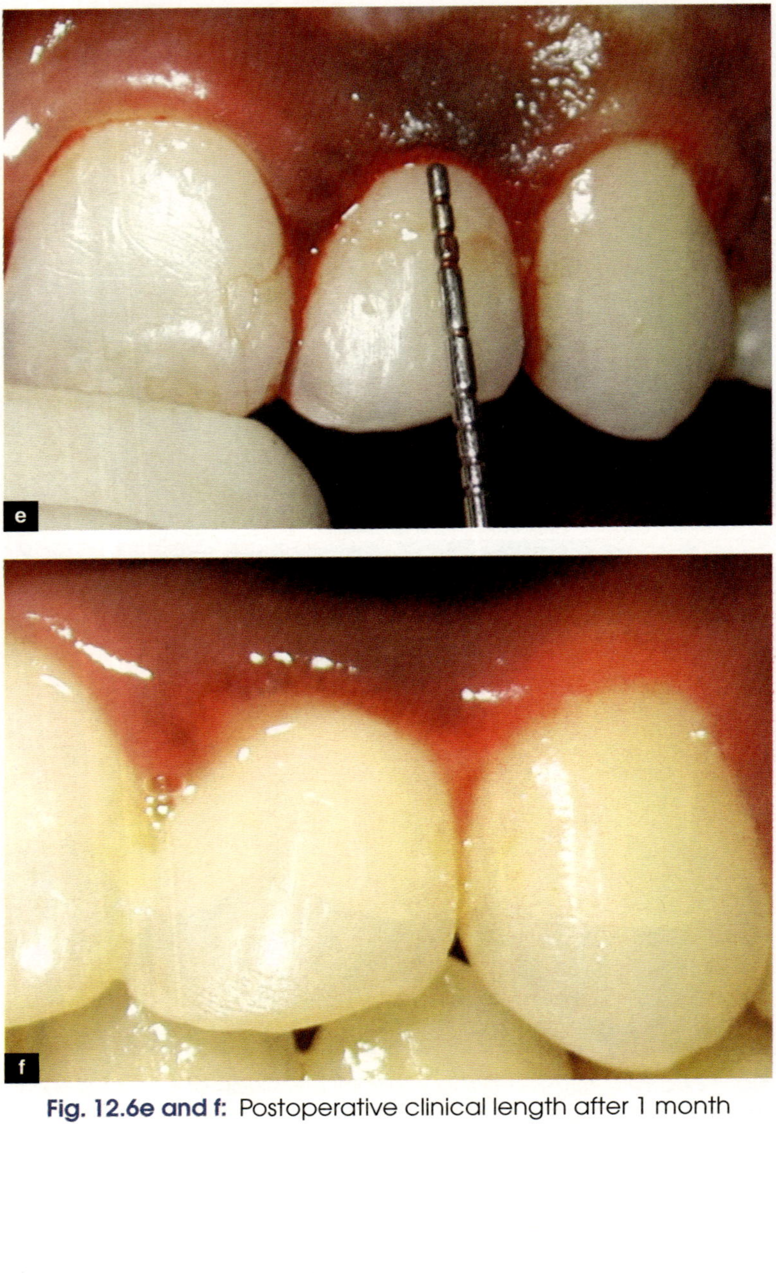

Fig. 12.6e and f: Postoperative clinical length after 1 month

Labial Frenectomy (Fig. 12.7a to f)

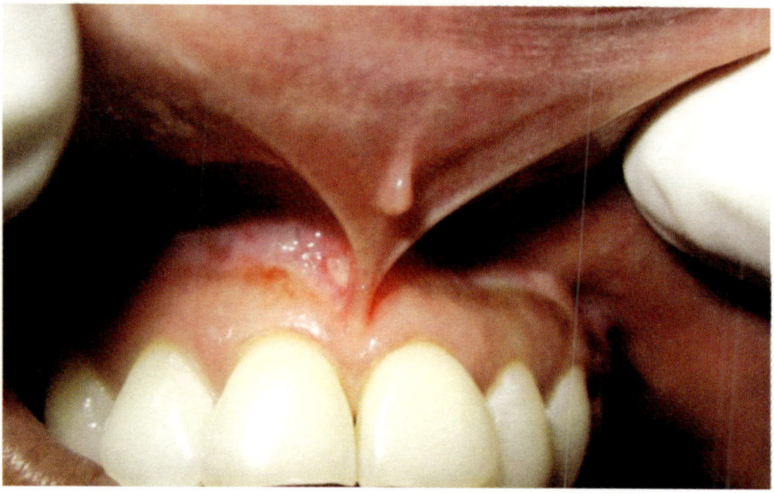

Fig. 12.7a: Preoparative frontal view

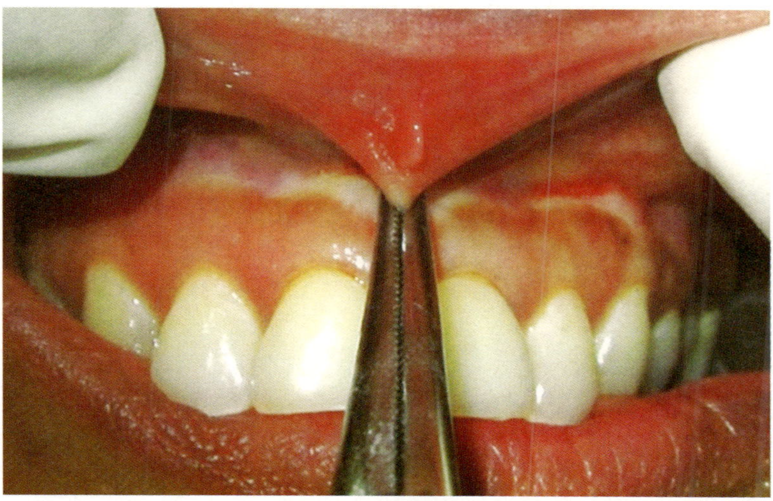

Fig. 12.7b: Frenum held with a hemostat

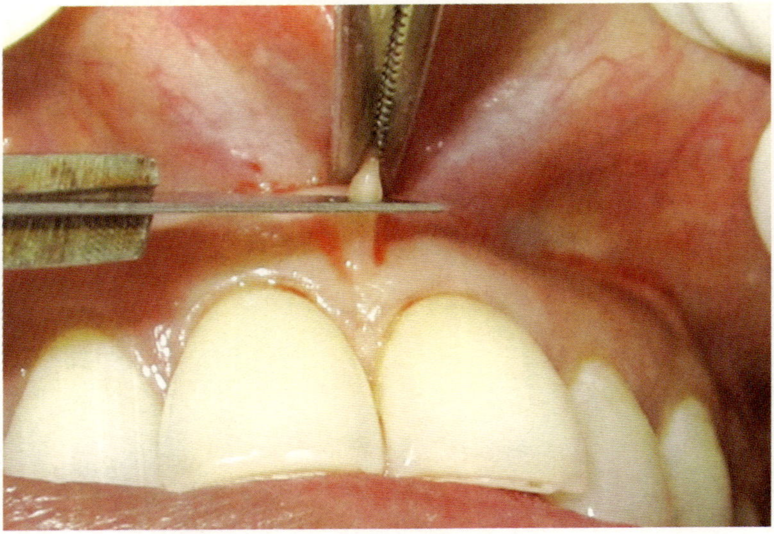

Fig. 12.7c: Incision

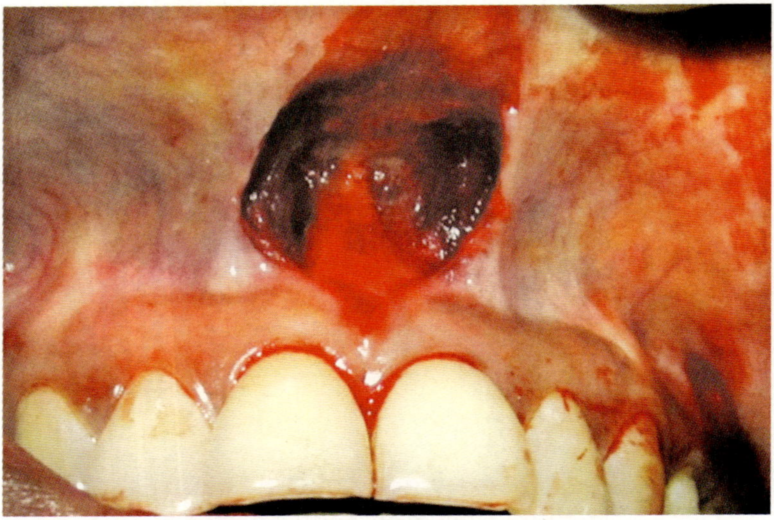

Fig. 12.7d: Frenectomy

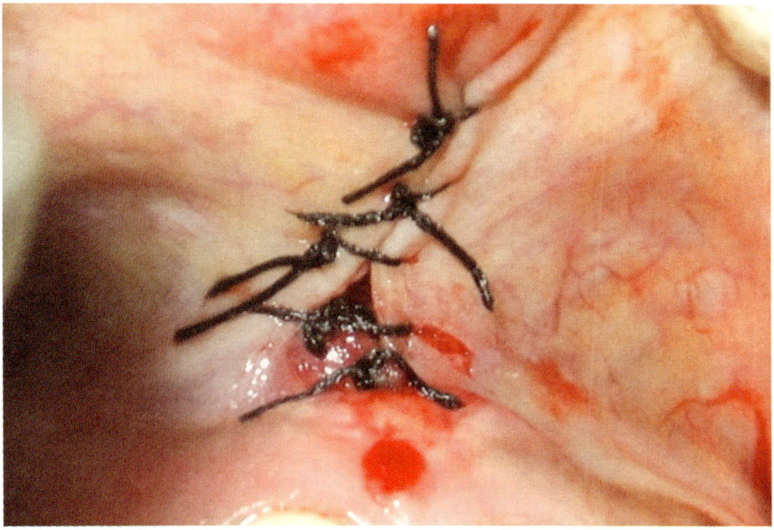

Fig. 12.7e: Single interrupted sutures

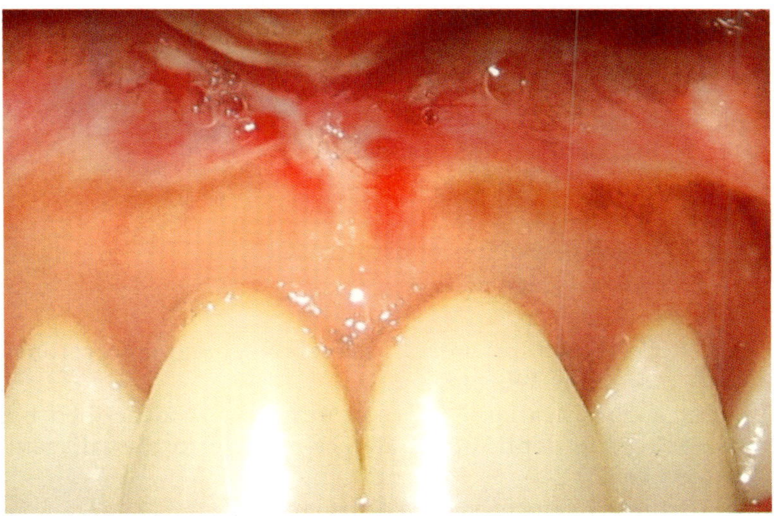

Fig. 12.7f: Postoperative after 1 month

13

Ridge Augmentation

Ridge augmentation procedures refer to surgical procedures that permit us to reconstruct the deformed ridge.

Consequences of a deficient ridge

1. Unappealing emergence profile,
2. Inadequate root eminence,
3. Long pontics to compensate for the ridge defect,
4. Empty gingival embrasures resulting in black triangles,
5. Inability to maintain adequate oral hygiene.

A. Classification of ridge defects

1. Seiberts classification (1983)
   a. Class I defect
      1. Buccolingual loss of tissue (B-L)
      2. Normal ridge height
   b. Class II defect
      1. Apicocoronal loss of tissue (A-C)
      2. Normal ridge width
   c. Class III defect
      - Combined loss in both buccolingual and apicocoronal direction (B-L and A-C)
2. Allen's classification—Ridge deformity was described by assessing the depth of the defect relative to the adjacent ridge.
   a. **Type A:** Apicocoronal loss of ridge contour
   b. **Type B:** Buccolingual loss of ridge contour
   c. **Type C:** Combined loss of apicocoronal and bucco-lingual ridge contour
   d. **Mild:** Defect less than 3 mm

e. **Severe:** Defect greater than 6 mm
f. **Moderate:** Defect in between 3 and 6 mm

B. Measures for prevention of bone ridge collapse after tooth extraction are indicated in cases of (Borghetti and Laborde, 1996):

1. Fracture of the vestibular osseous plate during tooth extraction or due to trauma
2. Resorption of the vestibular osseous plate
3. Presence of a thin vestibular bone plate.

C. Classification of ridge augmentation procedures

1. Soft tissue procedures:
1a. Pedicle graft procedure: Roll flap procedures
1b. Free graft procedures:
 i. Pouch graft procedure
 ii. Interpositional graft procedure
 iii. Onlay graft procedure.
2. Hard tissue procedures: Bone grafting
3. Guided bone regeneration
4. Sinus lift procedures
5. Distraction osteogenesis
 a. Ridge splitting
 b. Controlled tissue expansion

D. Surgical techniques

1. *Roll flap procedure (Abrams, 1980)* (*Fig. 13.1*)

Indications

a. Treatment of small to moderate class I ridge defects, primarily in cases with a single-tooth space.
b. Augments tissue apically and labially to the cervical area of a pontic
c. To enhance the appearance of normal tooth gingiva interface at recipient site.

2. *Pouch graft procedures*

Indications: The technique is used to correct class I defects.

Technique: A subepithelial pouch is prepared in the area of the ridge deformity, into which a free graft of connective tissue is placed and molded to create the desired contour of the ridge. The

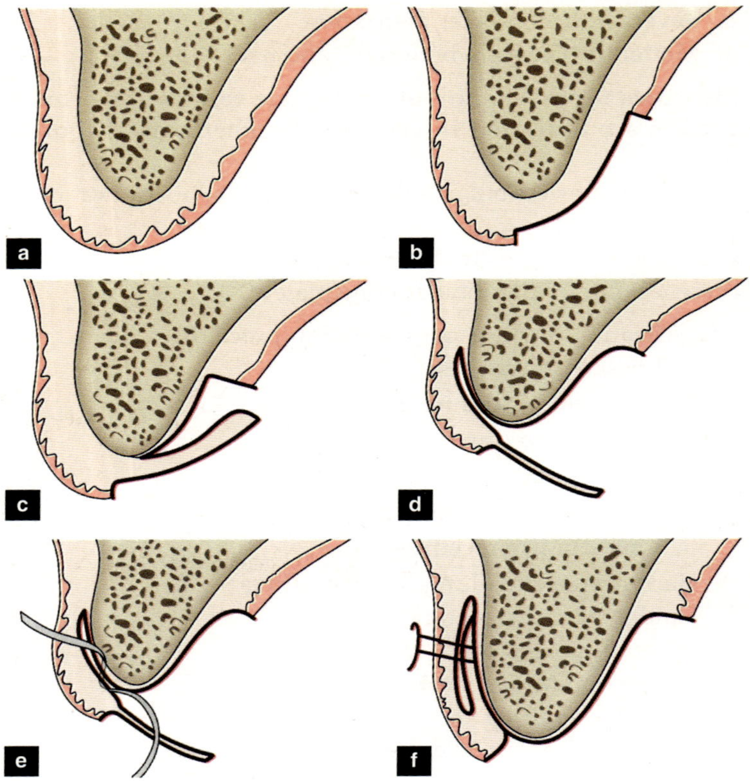

Fig. 13.1a to f: Roll flap procedure. (a) Cross-section of residual ridge prior to treatment; (b) Removal of epithelium; (c) The elevation of pedicle; (d) Pouch is created; (e) Sutures are placed at mucogingival junction to catch the pedicle flap and place it into the pouch; (f) Flap is secured and ridge convexity is created

entrance incision and the plane of dissection may be made in different ways:

a. *Coronal-apically:* The horizontal incision is made on the palatal or lingual side of the defect and the plane of dissection carried in an apical direction.
b. *Apical-coronally:* The horizontal incision is made high in the vestibule near the mucobuccal fold and the plane of dissection is carried coronally to the crest of the ridge.

c. Laterally: One or two vertical entrance incisions are started from either side of the defect. The plane of dissection is made laterally across the span of the deformity.

3. ***Interpositional graft procedure (Fig. 13.2)***

Indications: It is indicated in correction of class I as well as small and moderate class II defects.

Technique (Seibert, 1991): Interpositional grafts are not completely submerged and are covered in the manner that a subepithelial connective tissue graft is placed. Therefore, there is no need to remove the epithelium from the surface of the donor tissue.

4. ***Onlay graft procedures (Fig. 13.3)***

Indications: The Onlay procedure was designed to augment ridge defects in the apicocoronal plane, i.e. to gain ridge height. These are indicated in treatment of large Class II and class III defects.

Technique (Meltzer, 1979; Seibert, 1983)*:* Onlay grafts are epithelialized free grafts which, following placement; receive their nutrition from the de-epithelialized connective tissue of the recipient site.

GBR in Implant Therapy

There are two approaches to GBR in implant therapy

a. Simultaneous approach implant placement and GBR are performed simultaneously to create increased bone around the implant.
b. Staged approach GBR is used to increase the alveolar ridge or improve ridge morphology before implant placement which is placed after healing.

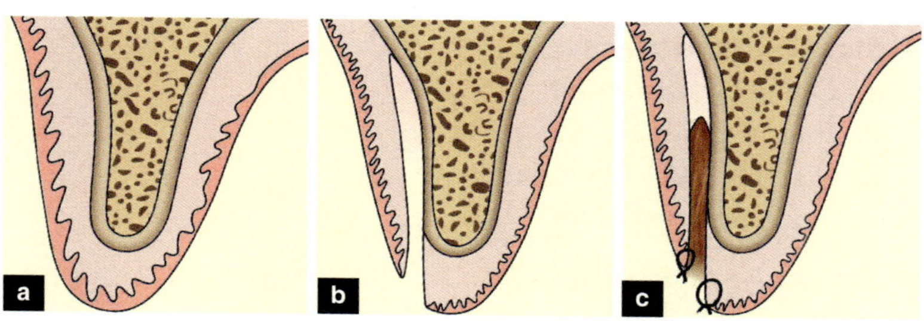

Fig. 13.2: Interpositional graft technique. (a) Class I ridge defect; (b) Labial partial thickness flap elevated to create the pouch; (c) A wedge shaped graft is flushed against the soft tissue in the pouch and sutured

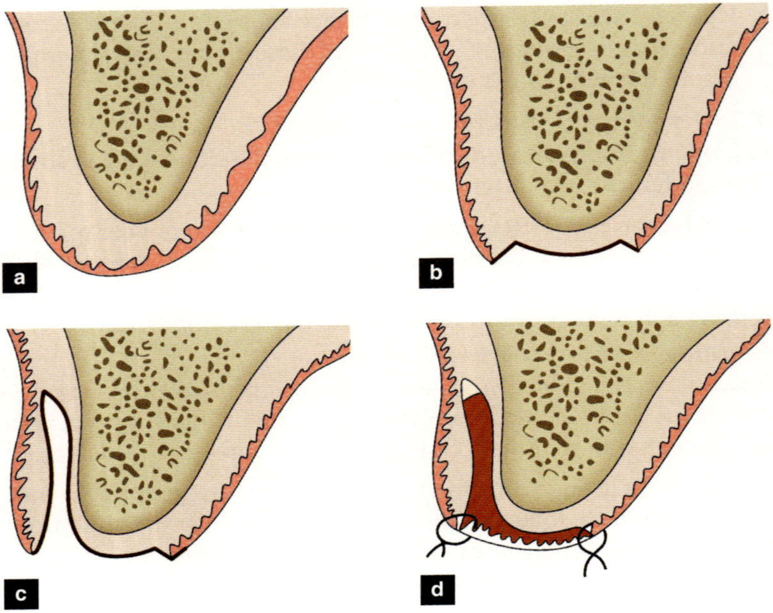

Fig. 13.3a to d: Onlay interpositional graft procedure. (a) Class III ridge defect; (b) Epithelium is removed on the labial-crestal side of the ridge to prepare the recipient bed for the onlay segment of the graft; (c) Partial-thickness dissection was then used to create a pouch for the interpositional section of the graft; (d) Graft sutured into position

Ridge Augmentation in Completely Edentulous Jaw

A. *Maxillary augmentation*

1. Onlay bone grafting
2. Inter positional bone grafts
3. Maxillary HA augmentation
4. Sinus lifts procedure

B. *Mandibular augmentation*

1. Superior border augmentation
2. Inferior border augmentation
3. HA augmentation of the mandible
4. GBR (osteopromotion)

Lateral Ridge Augmentation (Fig. 13.4a to i)

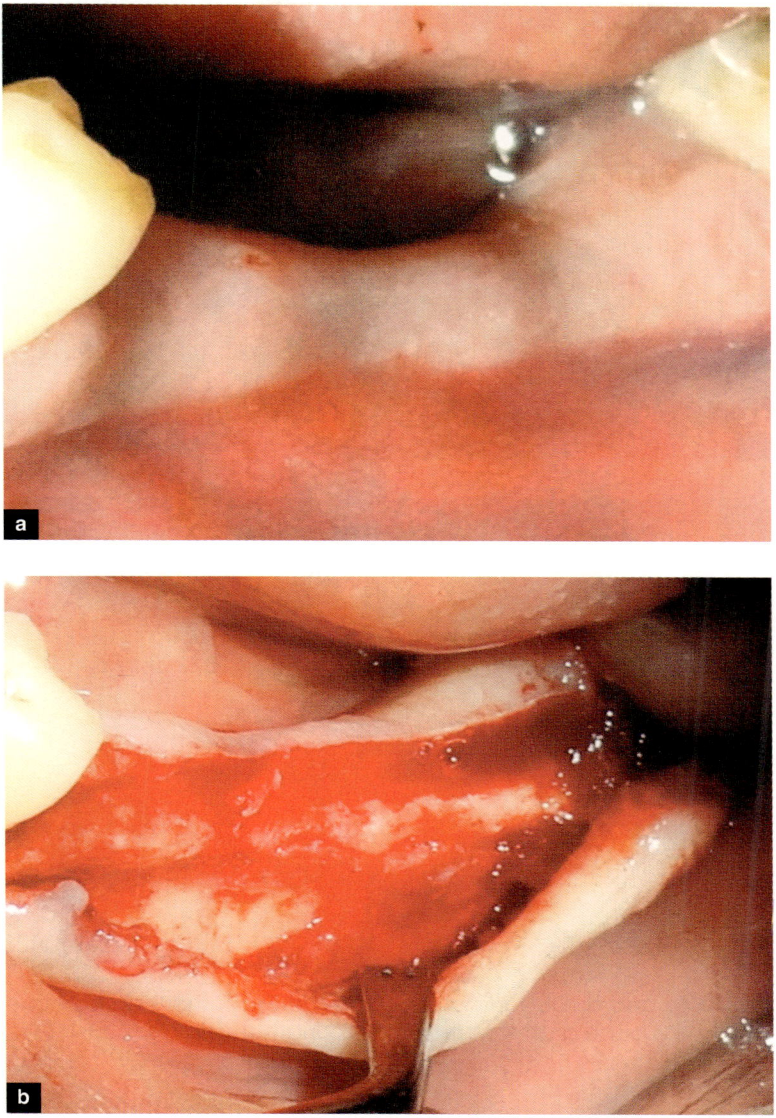

Fig. 13.4a and b: Preoperative 35, 36, 37-ridge augmentation site. Raising the mucoperiosteal flap

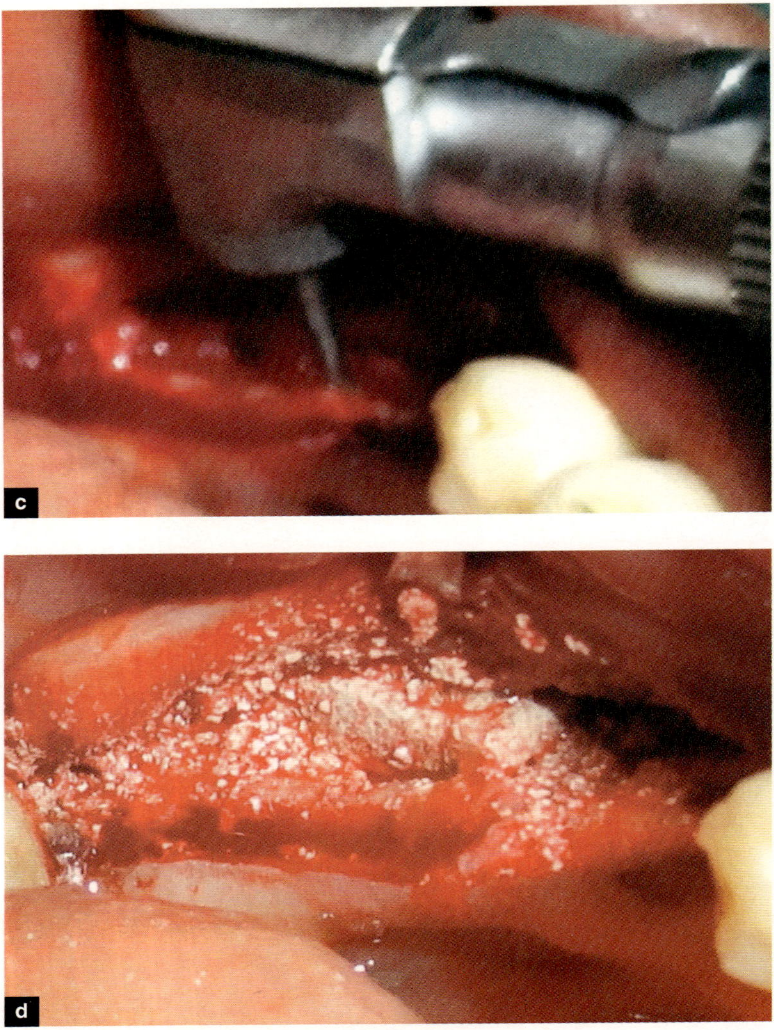

Fig. 13.4c and d: Decortication of the site. Placement of the bone block with bone graft for lateral ridge augmentation

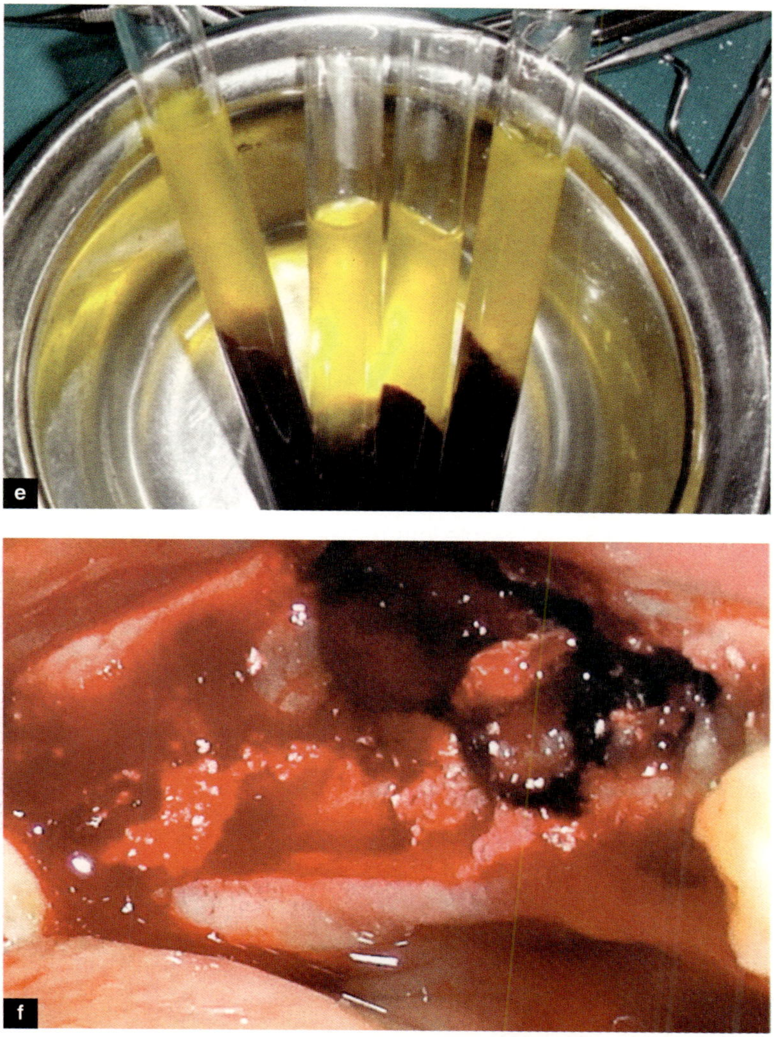

Fig. 13.4e and f: PRF procured and placed at the site for enhanced soft tissue healing and bone augmentation

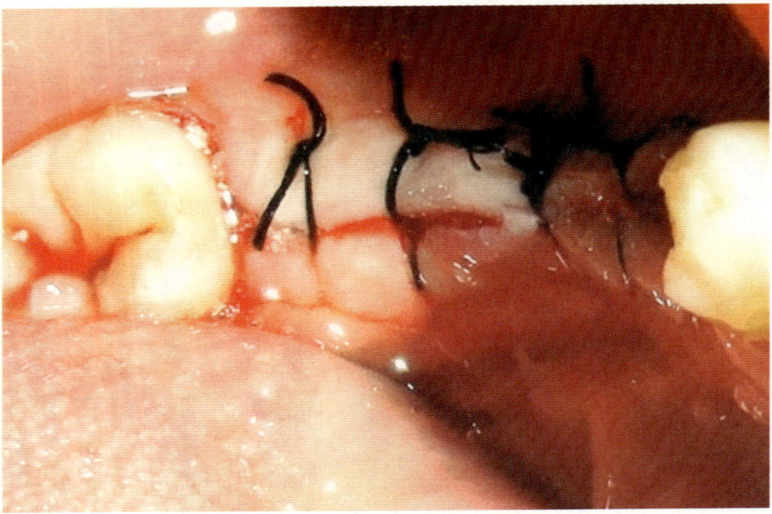

Fig. 13.4g: Single interrupted sutures placed

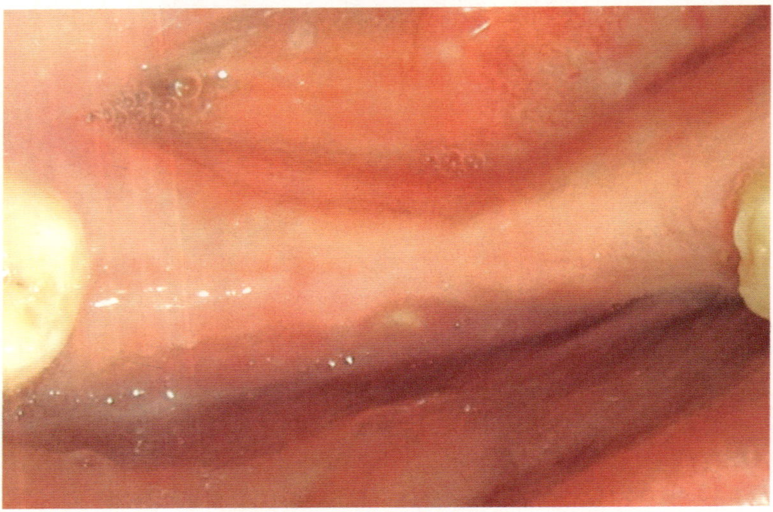

Fig. 13.4h: Postoperative after 3 months shows lateral augmentation

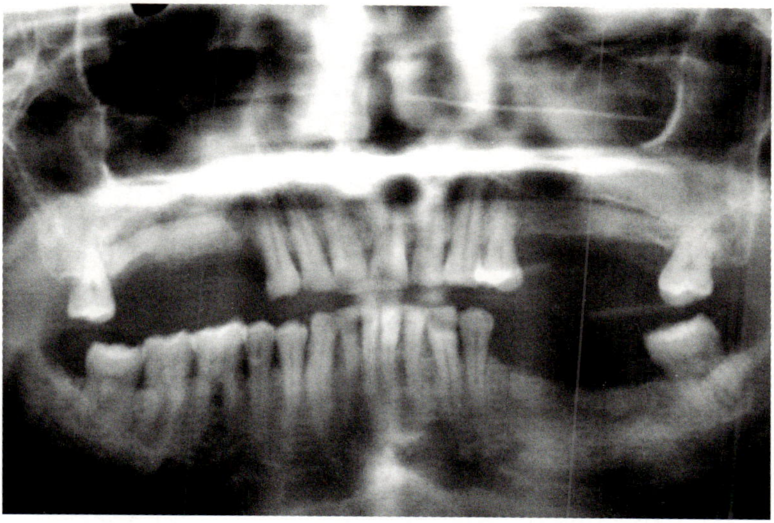

Fig. 13.4i: Postoperative OPG shows the presence of calcium hydroxyapatite bone blocks even after 3 months

14

Sutures and Suturing Techniques

SUTURES

A thread that either approximates or maintains tissues until the natural healing process has provided a sufficient level of wound strength. Also it compresses blood vessels in order to stop bleeding.

Table 14.1

Suture material	*Absorbable*	*Non-absorbable*
Mono-filament	• Surgical gut plain and chromic • Collagen plain and chromic • Monocryl • PDS II • Polyglactin 910	• Polyamide • Polypropylene • Stainless steel • Polyester
Multi-filament	• Polyglycolic acid • Polyglactin 910 • Polyglactin 910 rapide	• Surgical silk, surgical linen, cotton, stainless steel • Polyamide braided, Polyester braided • Polyester braided coated

Clinical Note

Most common nonresorbable sutures used today are expanded polytetrafluoroethylene, synthetic, monofilament suture. Most commonly used resorbable sutures are plain and chromic gut sutures.

Chromic sutures: Processed with chromic salts to make sutures resistant to enzymatic resorption.

Note: *Wicking effect refers to the ingress of bacteria from the oral cavity in the deeper areas of the wound, drawn through sutures. Monofilament sutures alleviate this effect.*

Suture Needles

A. Parts of Suture Needle (Fig. 14.1a and b)

1. *Eye:* It can be closed eye, French eye, swaged eye. Usually swaged (eyeless)
2. *Body:* Grasping area is the widest region. Body can be round, oval, rectangular, trapezoid, side flattened, curved, straight, half-curve, 5/8 circle, 1/2 circle, 3/8 circle, 1/4 circle.

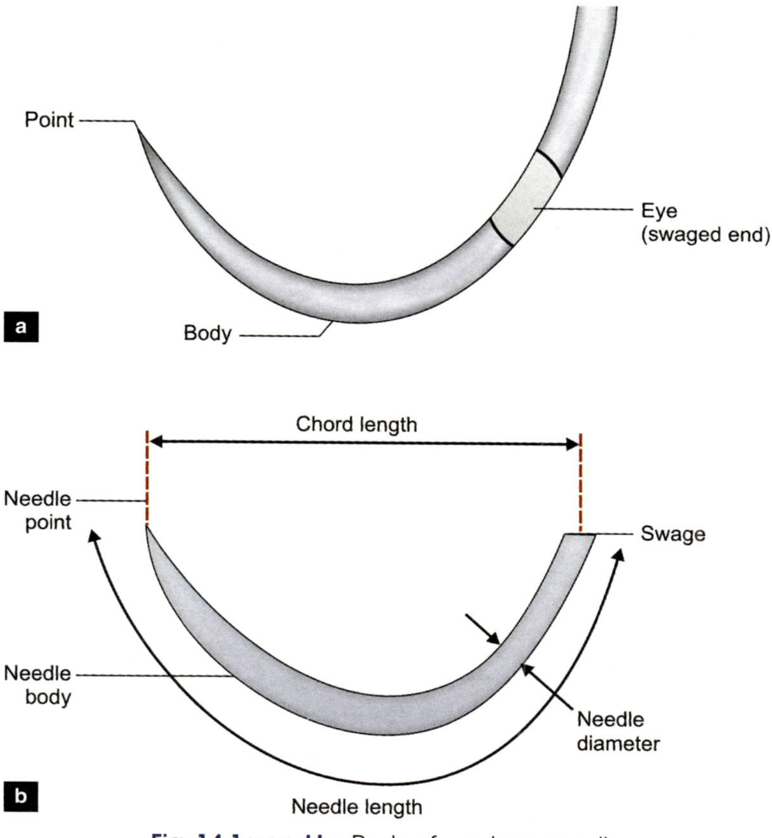

Fig. 14.1a and b: Parts of a suture needle

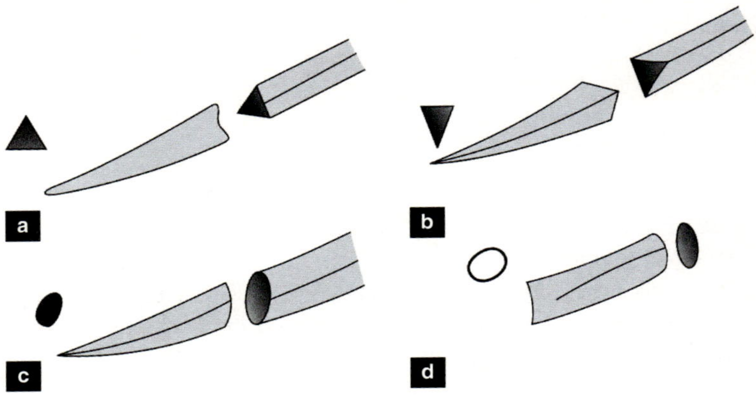

Fig. 14.2a to d: Classification of needle based on types of point. (a) Conventional cutting needle; (b) Reverse cutting needle; (c) Taper needle; (d) Smooth/blunt needle

3. *Point (Fig. 14.2):* Runs from tip to maximum cross-sectional area of body. It can be conventional, reverse cutting, taper, blunt.
4. *Needle length:* The distance measured along the needle itself from point to end.
5. *Radius:* The distance from the center of the circle to the body of the needle if the curvature of the needle were continued to make a full circle.

Clinical Note

Most common used sutures in oral cavity: Semicircular 3/8 or 5/8. The most common needle point preferred in periodontal surgeries is reverse cutting (prevents tearing of tissues).

Example of needle holders: Ochsner/Gile Wood model, Mayo Hegar, Castroviejo, Adson.

B. Principles of Suturing

a. The needle holder should grasp the needle at approximately 3/4 of the distance from the point (Fig. 14.3).
b. The needle should enter the tissue perpendicular to the surface.
c. The needle should be passed through the tissue following the curve of the needle.
d. The suture should be placed at an equal distance (2–3 mm) from the incision on both sides and at an equal depth.

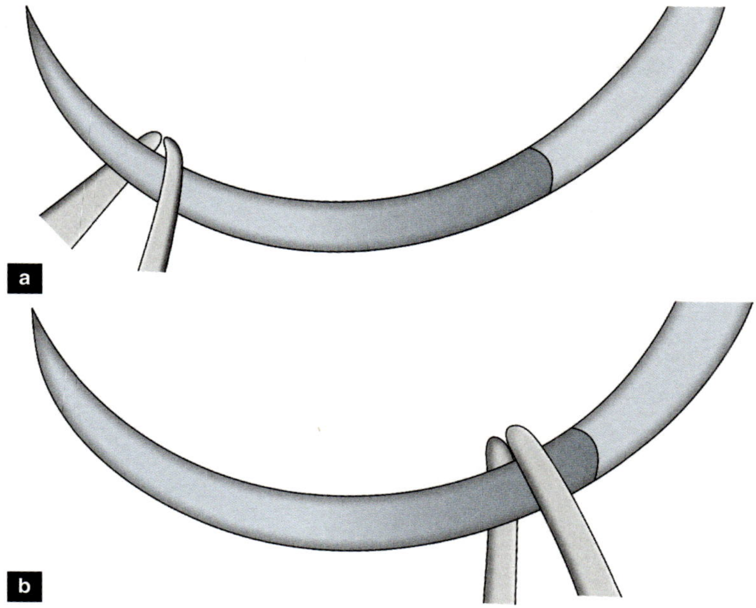

Fig. 14.3a and b: (a) Incorrect method of holding the needle; (b) Correct method of holding the needle at 3/4th distance from the point

e. The needle should be passed from the free to the fixed side.
f. The needle should be passed from the thinner to the thicker side.
g. The needle should be passed from the deeper to the superficial side.
h. The distance that the needle is passed into the tissue should be greater than the distance from the tissue edge.
i. Sutures should be placed approximately 3 to 4 mm apart.
j. Occasionally, extra tissue may be present on one side of the incision and cause a dog ear to be formed in the final phase of wound closure. Simply extending the length of the incision to hide the excess will produce an unsatisfactory result.

C. Suturing Techniques

a. *Interrupted:* Figure of eight, circumferential, mattress vertical and horizontal, intrapapillary, cross, laurel-loop.
b. *Continuous:* Papillary sling, vertical mattress, locking, anchor.

Table 14.2: Technique and indications

Technique	*Indications*
Interrupted	Closure of vertical releasing incisions and interproximal areas; replaced and coronally positioned flap closure
Sling	Allows separate facial or lingual flap positioning in isolated areas
Continuous sling	Single suture to close sextant or quadrant, facial and lingual flaps closed independently
Vertical	Narrow interdental spaces
Horizontal	Wider interdental spaces
Cross	Closure of vertical releasing incision
Anchoring	Guided tissue regeneration or bone grafts when an adjacent edentulous space is present, achieves primary closure
Laurel loop	Used in guided tissue regeneration

Knot (Fig. 14.4)

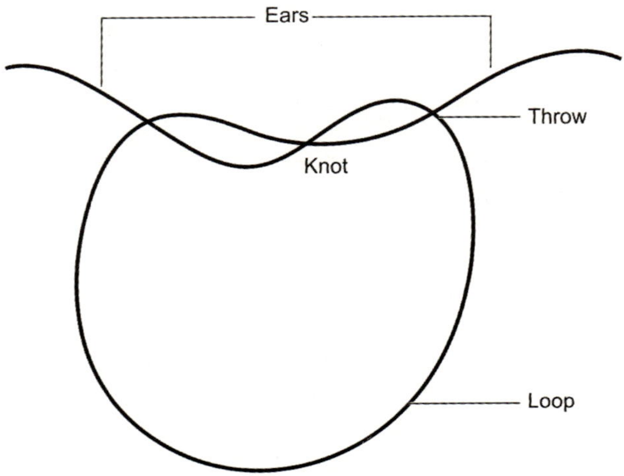

Fig. 14.4: Parts of a knot

Tissue approximation during healing depends on the knot stability.

Types of knot (Fig. 14.5)

1. Square knot
2. Surgeon's knot
3. Granny's knot

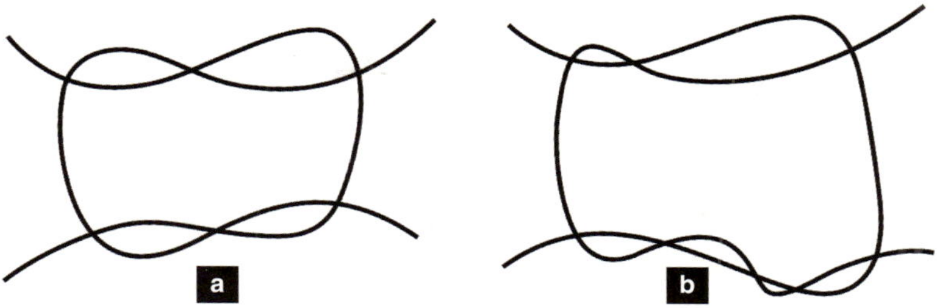

Fig. 14.5a and b: (a) Square knot; (b) Surgeon's knot

Clinical Note for Technique

1. Knot should be small and ends should be short, approximately 2–3 mm.
2. Knot should be tied firm, but not tight enough to cause blanching of the tissue.
3. Knot should never be tied on the incision line. It impairs healing.
4. Loose ends of thread at knot ends should be trimmed.
5. Suture removal should be done as atraumatically as possible.
6. Area should be cleaned with antiseptic/alcohol swab prior to suture removal.

Note: *Suture track is a separate wound and incites the same phenomena as in healing of the primary wound. Sometimes the suture track gets infected (stitch abscess), or the epithelial cells persist in the track (implantation or epidermal cysts).*

Alternatives to suturing: Staples, surgical zipper, adhesive tapes, clips and adhesives.

15

Endo Perio Continuum

The term perio-endo lesion has been used to describe lesions due to inflammatory products found in varying degrees in both periodontal and pulpal tissues (Simring and Goldberg in 1964).

Pathways of Communication (Fig. 15.1)

1. *Apical foramen:* Principal and most direct route of communication.
2. Lateral and accessory canals
3. *Dentinal tubules:* In root, tubules extend from pulp to dentinocemental junction. Diameter of tubules decreases with age and in response to continuous low grade stimuli.
4. *Developmental grooves:* Palatogingival grooves.
5. Enamel projections or pearls
6. Empty spaces created by destroyed sharpeys fibers
7. *Vertical root fracture:* Deep periodontal pocketing and localized destruction of the alveolar bone.
8. Perforation creates communication between root canal system and periodontal ligament.
9. *Resorption (internal/external):* Condition associated with either a physiologic or a pathologic process resulting in a loss of dentin, cementum and/or bone.

Clinical Note

Lateral canals: Perpendicular to the main canal.

Accessory canals: Branch off and run parallel to the main canal. Majority is found apically, with little prevalence in the middle and cervical root segments.

Charcot Leyden crystals: Crystals derived from the intracellular granules of eosinophils and basophils. These can be detected within a periapical lesion that failed to resolve after conventional endodontic treatment.

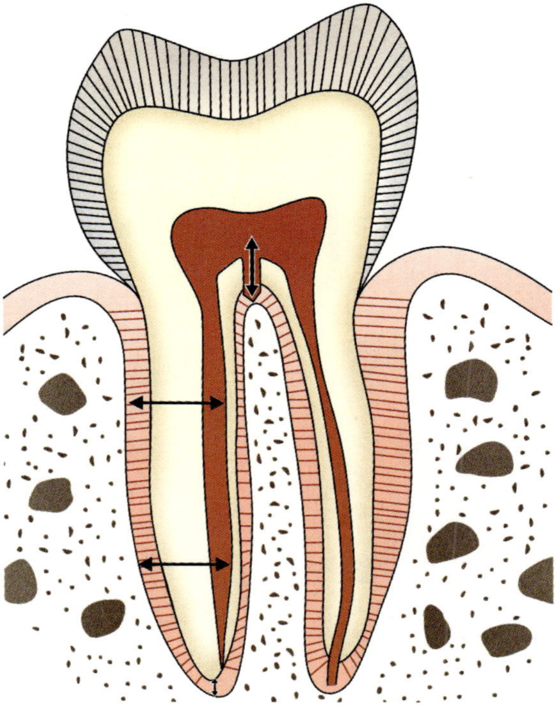

Fig. 15.1: Pathways of communication—apical foramen, lateral canal and accessory canals

Classification

A. Based on Etiology (Simon, Glick and Frank, 1972) (Fig. 15.2)

1. Primary endo
2. Primary perio
3. Secondary endo
4. Secondary perio
5. Combined lesion

B. Based on Etiology and Type of Therapy (Frank S. Weine, 1972)

Class I: Symptoms clinically and radiographically simulate periodontal disease, but are in fact due to pulpal inflammation and/or necrosis.

Class II: Both pulpal and periodontal disease concomitantly.

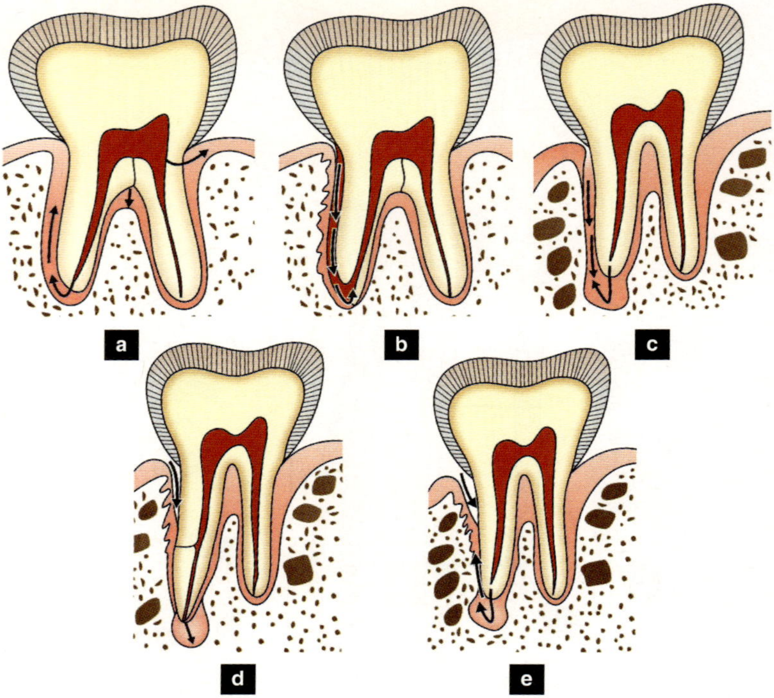

Fig. 15.2a to e: Classification by Simon, Glick and Frank. (a) Primary endo; (b) Primary perio; (c) Secondary perio; (d) Secondary endo; (e) Combined lesion

Class III: No pulpal problem but requires endodontic therapy plus root amputation to gain periodontal healing.

Class IV: Clinically and radiographically simulates pulpal or periapical disease but in fact has periodontal disease.

C. Abbott's Classification

1. Without communication

Infected root canal with some form of apical periodontitis and marginal periodontal disease with pocketing. No communication.

Clinically: Probing does not extend to periapical lesion.

Radiographically, bone can be seen between and separating, the periapical radiolucency and base of the pocket.

Clinical Note

Toothblushing *refers to vascular stasis and haemorrhage in the subodontoplastic vascular plexus caused by extreme heat generated in dry tooth preparation (Lindhe, 3rd ed).*

Increase in temperature by 5–6° is capable of inducing necrotic changes in pulp.

2. With communication

Clinically: Pocketing extends to the periapical lesion such that the periapical and periodontal diseases communicate with each other.

Radiographically: Appears as radiolucency and no bone can be seen

Diagnosis

1. *Visual examination:* Presence of inflammation, ulcerations, or sinus tracts. Teeth-caries, defective restorations, erosions, abrasions, cracks, fractures, and discolorations. Fractures should always be ruled out with transillumination and with radiographs taken at two different angles.
2. *Palpation and percussion:* Active periradicular inflammatory process creates hot zones. These elicit painful response to digital pressure.
3. *Mobility:* Mobility can be seen in periodontal lesions due to bone loss and in cases on endodontic lesions in cases of fractured tooth, if associated with secondary periodontal involvement.
4. *Pulp vitality testing:* Abnormal response—degenerative changes in the pulp, nonvital tooth in pulpal involvement.
5. *Pocket probing:* Important test to be performed when attempting to differentiate between endodontic and periodontal disease.

Note: *Retrograde periodontitis is a feature of endodontic lesions (lesions are narrow coronally than at apex. It is associated with deep but narrow pocket that can be traced with gutta percha. In true periodontal lesion, orthograde/marginal periodontitis is seen (lesion extends from Crestal gingival tissues till the apex of the root).*

Clinical Note

In a clinical scenario differentiating between pain, abscesses due to periodontal and pulpal reasons requires major attention to be a successful practitioner.

Patient's history, symptoms, clinical and radiographic signs help in making a decision.

Symptoms: *Complaint of acute/intermittent/chronic pain. Type of pain: Localized/Radiating/dull gnawing pain. Differentiate between pulpal and periodontal lesions.*

Sensitivity to thermal stimuli—differentiating between reversible and irreversible pulpitis.

Patients' response to percussion, palpation, biting, vitality testing and pocket probing*—Periradicular lesions cause more pain on pressure, percussion and palpation (bony plate is involved in extreme cases) as compared to periodontal lesion (no involvement of periosteum).*

Signs: *Edema, redness and swelling in periradicular lesion is mostly confined at root apex compared to cervical location in periodontal abscess.*

Suppuration *in periodontal abscess will be mostly evident during probing. In periradicular lesion, pus discharge will be seen through a sinus or at some distance from site of infection.*

Radiographically: *Coronal status, lesion appearance (at apex or cervical), extent of bone loss should be evaluated. Periradicular radiolucency (PARL) is seen in retrograde periodontitis.*

Treatment Strategies

1. *Primary endodontic lesion:* Root canal treatment is the ideal treatment modality.
2. *Primary endodontic lesions with secondary periodontal involvement:* Root canal treatment, periodontal treatment. Prognosis dependent on ability to treat both disease entities. Periodontal healing occurs after a successful pulpal treatment.
3. *Secondary periodontal lesion:* Periodontal therapy followed by guided tissue regeneration, root amputation. Prognosis depends on outcome of periodontal therapy, extent of periodontitis and patients ability to comply with long term treatment and maintenance therapy.
4. *Primary periodontal lesions with secondary endodontic involvement:* Periodontal therapy, root amputation, guided tissue regeneration. Prognosis dependent on periodontal treatment and further root canal treatment.
5. *True combined lesion:* Endodontic therapy, periodontic therapy, hemisection, bicuspidization, root amputation. Prognosis depends on outcome of periodontal therapy. Better prognosis with primary pulpal lesion and with short-term lesion.

6. *Concomitant pulpal and periodontal lesion:* Both entities must be treated concomitantly. Prognosis dependent on removal of individual causes.

Pulpal Periodontal Syndrome

Defined as one involving inflammation/degeneration of the pulp with clinical pocket on same tooth and can be initiated by either pulpal or periodontal disease. Particularly true in molar teeth.

Author's Note

Treatment of endo perio lesion poses a dilemma for the clinician.

History is of utmost point in arriving at diagnosis. History of periodontal treatment (Lodged calculus, failed treatment), previous endodontic treatment should always be taken first.

Symptoms and signs mentioned in text should be noticed with keen eye.

A treatment plan should be charted and enough time should be allowed for the tissues to heal.

16

Periodontal–Restorative Interrelationship

Rationale for Establishing Periodontal Health Prior to Restorative Procedures

1. Establishment of sound tooth margins prior to tooth preparation.
2. Adequate tooth length for retention, access for tooth preparation and impression making to prevent failure of the prosthesis.
3. Restorations on teeth free of inflammation tend to be more stable and comfortable to the patient.
4. Orthodontic procedures completed without prior periodontal treatment (if indicated) tend to result in negative changes that complicate further maintenance.

Note: *A period of 4 weeks should be provided to determine soft tissue and pocket depth changes after Phase I of periodontal therapy. A period of 2 months of healing should be allowed after soft tissue grafting procedures prior to restorative procedures.*

Preprosthetic Surgical Procedures

1. Crown lengthening procedures
2. Preservation of ridge morphology after tooth extraction
3. Management of mucogingival problems

A. Biological Considerations

1. *Biological width (Fig. 16.1)*
   a. *Biologic width evaluation:* Biological width is defined as physiological dimension of junctional epithelium and connective tissue attachment. Average biological width is 2 mm.
   b. Determined accurately by transgingival probing/sounding (distance between bone and the restoration margin

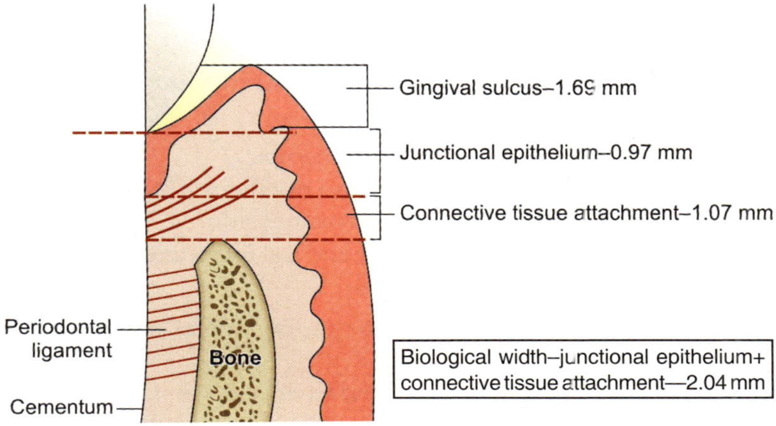

Fig. 16.1: Dimensions of biologic width

determined through the anesthetized tissue with the periodontal probe).

c. *Biological width violation:* Distance less than 2 mm at one or more locations determines biological width violation. It results in bone loss, gingival recession, gingival inflammation and pocket formation depending on the gingival biotype and the bone anatomy.
d. *Correction of violation:* Surgically by removing bone away from proximity to the restoration margin or orthodontically extruding the tooth and moving the margins away from bone.

Clinical Note

1. *A highly scalloped thin gingiva is more prone to recession. Pocket formation is more common in flat periodontium with thick fibrous tissue.*
2. *At least 2–3 mm of clinical space should be present between alveolar bone and tooth margin to establish gingival health.*
3. ***If the patient experiences pain while clinician is exploring the margins of the crown restoration, it is a definitive indication of biologic width violation.***
4. *Another sign of biologic width violation after crown placement is patient's symptoms of pain and signs of gingival redness, inflammation after few days of restoration.*
5. *Transgingival probing to determine sulcus depth and casts should be correlated to determine the required distance between margin and bone.*

Indications of Surgical crown lengthening (Carranza):

1. Subgingival caries/fracture
2. Inadequate clinical crown length for retention
3. Unaesthetic gingival contour

Indications of orthodontic extrusion (Carranza):

1. Gingival tissue contour is correct but there is biologic width violation on the facial/interproximal side.

   There are two techniques: Slow and fast orthodontic extrusion.
2. Margin placement guidelines

Crown margin placements can be supragingival, equigingival, subgingival.

Supragingival is most preferred and have the last impact on periodontium. The greatest biological risk occurs with subgingival margins.

a. Rules to determine margin placement (Fig. 16.2)
   1. Sulcus depth 1.5 mm or less-margin placed 0.5 mm below the tissue crest

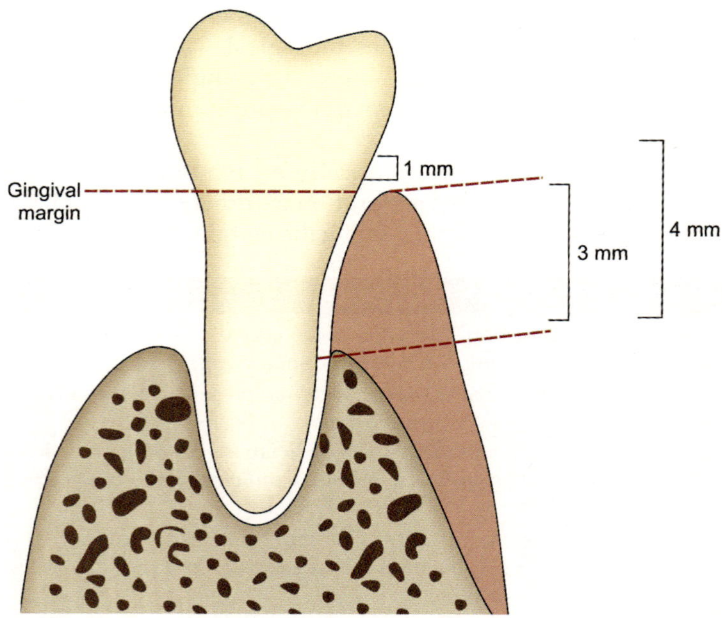

Fig. 16.2: At least 1mm of sound tooth structure should be provided above gingival margin for gingival health

2. Sulcus depth more than 1.5 mm margin placed half the depth of the sulcus below the tissue crest
3. Sulcus depth greater than 2 mm—gingivectomy performed to lengthen the tooth and create 1.5 mm sulcus. Later margin placement according to rule 1.

B. Aesthetic Tissue Management

1. Managing Interproximal embrasures (Fig. 16.3): An ideal Interproximal embrasure houses the gingiva papilla without impinging on it. It extends the interproximal contact to the tip of papilla so that no space exists to trap food and is aesthetically pleasing (Carranza, 9th ed).

   A harmonious relationship should be maintained between the interproximal papilla and the interproximal embrasure created

Note: *Papillary height is established by level of bone, biologic width and form of gingival embrasure.*
Interproximal sulcus depth is 1. 1.5 mm deeper than that on facial surface.
Embrasure of ideal width has a sulcus depth of 2.5–3 mm.

Clinical Note

1. *If bone under a papilla is apical to adjacent bone levels, then periodontal disease/bone loss is the cause of open embrasure in that area. Requires periodontal therapy.*
2. *However, if bone levels are at same level, then open embrasure is caused by embrasure form of the teeth.*

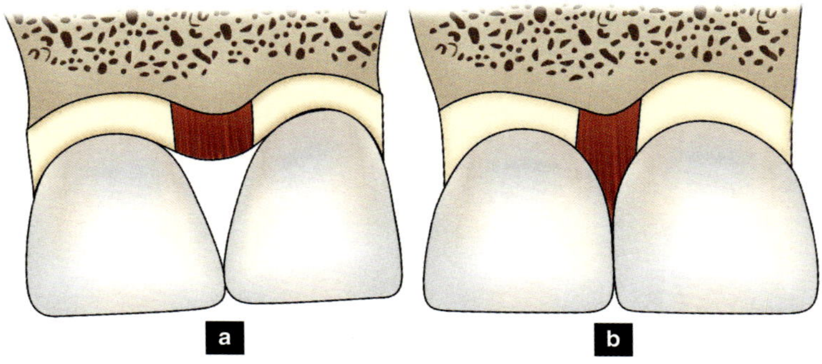

Fig. 16.3a and b: (a) Tapered tooth structure results in large gingival embrasure form; (b) Ideal tooth form with the same volume of gingival tissue, covering the top of attachment

Clinical Note

While placing an ovate pontic, three points should be considered

1. *Ridge height needs to match the height of the interproximal papilla,*
2. *The gingival margin height must be at the same level,*
3. *Ridge tissue must be facial to the ideal cervical facial form of pontic, so that pontic can emerge from tissue.*

by restorations. If the embrasure is too narrow, papilla grows out of facial and lingual surface, forms a col and becomes inflamed.

Correcting open gingival embrasures restoratively and in patients with gingival recession:

a. Correcting open gingival embrasures due to shape of teeth. margins of the restoration are carried subgingivally by 1.0 to 1.5 mm. Emergence profile moves the contact point towards papilla. It is done with direct bonded restorations.
b. In posteriors since inter root width is greater, chances of overhangs exist with restorations.

2. *Pontic design:* There are four options in pontic design—ovate, sanitary, ridge lap and modified ridge lap (Figs 16.4 to 16.6). Clinical considerations in selecting optimal pontic design:
   a. Sanitary (Fig. 16.6) and ovate pontic have convex under surface easiest to clean

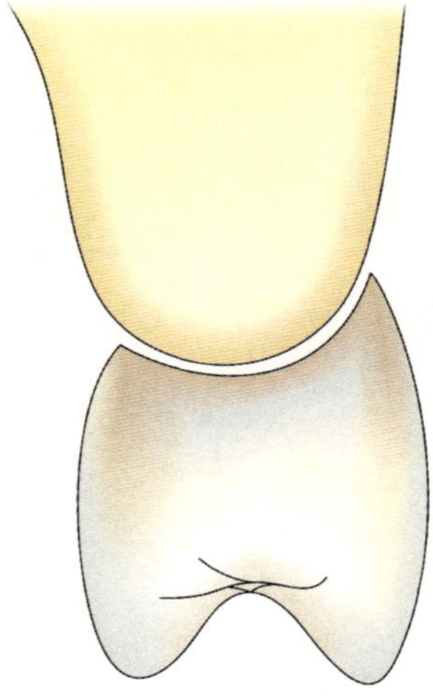

Fig. 16.4: Ridge lap pontic

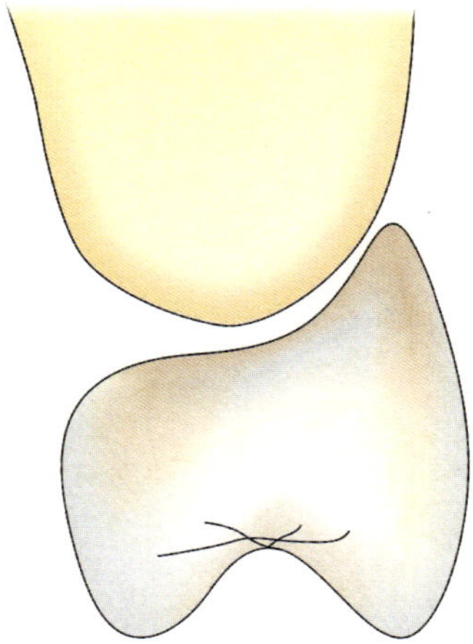

Fig. 16.5: Modified ridge lap pontic

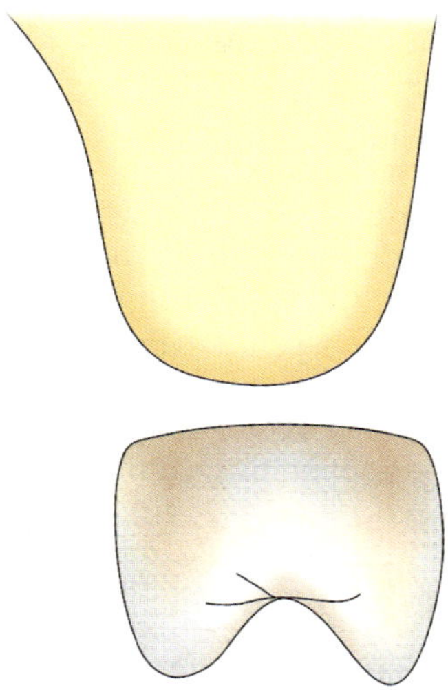

Fig. 16.6: Sanitary pontic

b. Ridge lap (Fig. 16.4) and modified ridge lap—concave surface and are difficult to access.
c. Ovate is the ideal pontic form (Fig. 16.7). In aesthetic area, receptor site is crated 1 to 1.5 mm below the tissue in the facial aspect.

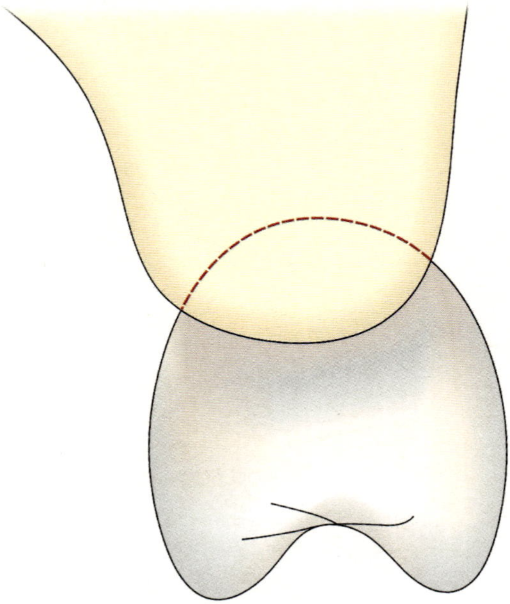

Fig. 16.7: Ovate pontic

An appearance of free gingival margin is created. In posteriors, facial portion of pontic is at same level of ridge. It produces a flat easily cleansable tissue surface.

d. Modified ridge lap pontic (Fig. 16.5): This is placed on extraction site, if inadequate ridge exists for ovate pontic. This pontic has the advantage of following the convexity on the facial surface, open lingual form allows adequate access for oral hygiene.

Author's Note

1. *Active periodontal infection and inflammation must be treated prior to aesthetic, restorative, orthodontic procedures.*
2. *A complex periodontal restorative interrelationship should be determined via casts, photographs, tactile sensitivity to determine tooth bone margin distance.*

17

Periodontal Plastic Microsurgery

DEFINITION

Microsurgery is defined as surgery performed under magnification of 10× or more, done under surgical microscope (Daniel, 1979).

Note: *The three elements, i.e. magnification, illumination, and instruments are called the microsurgical triad (Kim et al. 2001).*

Two basic types of magnification systems are commonly used: The surgical microscope and loupes:

Surgical microscope: It is a complicated system of lenses that allows stereoscopic vision at a magnification of approximately 440× with an excellent illumination of the working area.

The optical unit includes the following components:

1. Magnification changer
2. Objective lenses
3. Binocular tubes,
4. Eyepieces, and
5. Lighting unit

Loupes: These are fundamentally dual monocular telescopes with side by side lenses convergent to focus on operative field. This convergent lens optical system is called *Keplerian optical system.*

The loupes are further classified as:

1. Single-lens magnifiers (clip-on, flip-up, jewelers glasses) and
2. Multilens telescopic loupes (compound or prism loupes)

1. In periodontal surgery, magnifications of 45× for loupe spectacles and 10–20× for surgical microscopes appear to be ideal depending on the kind of intervention.

2. 12–15×—dealing with a localized problem such as the coverage of a single soft tissue recession or interdental wound closure after guided tissue regeneration of an infrabony defect.
3. 68×—for clinical inspections or surgical interventions when the entire quadrant is under operation.
4. 15–25×—are more likely limited to the visual examination of clinical details only, such as in endodontic interventions.

Advantages of loupes and microscopes

1. Improved visual acuity and precise handgrip—increase accuracy with enhance motor skill.
2. Minimal tissue trauma—smaller incisions and reduced surgical fields.
3. Primary passive wound closure—achieved by microsuturing to eliminate gaps and dead spaces at the wound edge.
4. Ergonomics, body posture and arm support are improved.
5. Titanium instruments and round handles permit precise rotation.

Disadvantage of loupes and microscopes

1. Increased expenses of the equipment
2. Extended learning phase for the surgeon and his assistant.

Note: *Surgical microscopes offer greater versatility, depth of focus, field of view and stability as compared to loupes.*

Microsurgical Instrumentation and Suturing Techniques

A basic set comprises a needle holder, microscissors, microscalpel holder, anatomic and surgical forceps, and a set of various elevators.

1. Monofilament suture material such as polypropylene or polydiaxanone. Suture size ranges from 6–0 to 9–0.
2. Swaged sutures; Tapered needles preferred. Needle diameter larger than suture size. Chord distance is an important determinant.
3. Needle should penetrate the tissue at 90 degree perpendicular to tissue surface and exit perpendicular to incision line.
4. Bite size is between 1 and 1.5 times the tissue thickness.
5. The distance between bite sizes on either side of the wound should be symmetrical. Multiple sutures should be placed to prevent stress breakage of sutures or tissue tearing.
6. Two basic knots—square knot or reef knot and English surgeon's knot. Reef knot has better internal stability than any other knot.

18

Piezoelectric Bone Surgery

Piezosurgery was invented by Vercellotti and developed by Mectron medical technology.

Piezosurgery is an electronic device that generates ultrasonic vibrations at variable frequency. The ultrasonic frequency is modulated from 10, 30, and 60 cycles/s (Hz) to 29 kHz. Low frequency enables cutting of mineralized structures, not soft issue.

The Piezosurgery tip vibrates within a range of 60–200 mm, which allows clean cutting with precise incisions.

Consists of piezoelectric ultrasonic transducer and variable cutting inserts.

Inserts Classified based on Functional and Clinic Characteristics

Functional classification: Sharp, smooth and blunt.

1. Sharp insert are for osteotomy and osteoplasty. Made of nitride titanium steel.
2. Smoothening inserts are diamond coated and is used to complete the cut near soft tissue.
3. Blunt inserts are characterized by rounded ends and are used to refine the cut in contact with soft tissue.

Clinical classification: OP, EX, IM.

1. OP is used to perform osteoplasty.
2. EX is used to perform extractions.
3. IM is used to perform implant site preparation.

Two operating modes: BONE (for cutting bone), ROOT (to shape, debride and smooth root surfaces).

a. Bone operating mode is low ultrasonic frequency for cutting small cortical and cancellous bone fragments.

b. Root operating mode is for scaling, root planning and root debridement. Intracanal debridement is also done by an ideal power level of ultrasonic frequency.

Clinical characteristics of piezoelectric surgery: Microprecision, selective cutting, maximum visibility, excellent healing.

Clinical Applications

1. *Periodontal surgeries:* Inserts easily detach the secondary flap and remove inflammatory granulation tissue. Ultrasonic vibrations act together with the cavitation of irrigation fluid. Ultrasound activates cellular response of healing mechanisms. Intraoperative time is reduced, thereby lessening complications.
2. *Minor surgical procedures:* Crown lengthening and gingivectomy
3. Implant site preparation
4. *Tooth extractions:* Less invasive technique, maintains the integrity of the alveolar bone.
5. *Regenerative surgeries:* Piezosurgery does not cause lamellar fracture of the bone, favors release of bone morphogenetic proteins, hence onset of osteogenesis at the wound site.
6. *Miscellaneous:* Ridge expansion, bone harvesting, and sinus lift.

Advantages: Low surgical trauma, fast healing of tissues, good control during surgery.

Note: *The piezoelectric instrument used for periodontal surgeries, tooth extractions, implant sinus lift operations work with an amplitude of 80 micrometer, and a frequency of 30,000 cycles/sec.*

19 LASERs (Light Amplification by Stimulated Emission of Radiations) in Periodontology

Theodore Maiman (1960)—First working laser red ruby laser.
First dental laser was marketed by Myers (1989).

Laser-tissue Interaction Results in Either of the Four Phenomenon

Scatter, absorption, reflection, transmission (refraction)
Effect of rise of tissue temperature (photothermal interaction).

Zones in Laser Irradiated Tissue

Carbonization (innermost), vaporization, coagulation, protein denaturation, stimulating zone (outermost)

Table 19.1	
37–50°C	• **Hyperthermia** • No destruction
60–70°C	• **Coagulation and protein denaturation** • Tissue whitens and blanches • Removal of granulation tissue
70–80°C	• **Welding** • Adherence of layers → stickiness of collagen
100–150°C	• **Vaporization and ablation** • Micro explosion → interstitial water in hard tissue is exploded → physical collapse of HA crystals → *spallation*
> 200°C	• **Carbonization** • Burnt and dehydrated tissue • Char layer formation → CO, cyanide and cyanates

Various Types of Lasers (Table 19.2)

Table 19.2

Laser type		*Wavelength*	*Color*
Excimer lasers	Argon fluoride (ArF)	193 nm	Ultraviolet
	Xenon chloride (XeCl) 308 nm		Ultraviolet
Gas lasers	Argon	488 nm 514 nm	Blue Blue-green
	Helium Neon (HeNe)	637 nm	Red
	Carbon dioxide (CO2)	10,600 nm	Infrared
Diode lasers	Indium Gallium Arsenide Phosphorus (InGaAsP)	655 nm 670–830 nm	Red Red-infrared
	Gallium Aluminum Arsenide (GaAlAs)	840 nm	Infrared
	Gallium Arsenide (GaAs)	980 nm	Infrared
	Indium Gallium Arsenide (InGaAs)		
Solid state lasers	Frequency-doubled Alexandrite	337 nm	Ultraviolet
	Potassium titanyl Phosphate (KTP)	532 nm	Green
	Neodymium:YAG (Nd:YAG)	1,064 nm	Infrared
	Holmium: YAG (Ho:YAG)	2,100 nm	Infrared
	Erbium, chromium: YSGG (Er, Cr: YSGG)	2,780 nm	Infrared
	Erbium: YSGG (Er: YSGG)	2,790 nm	Infrared
	Erbium: YAG (Er: YAG)	2,940 nm	Infrared

Applications of Lasers in Dentistry

1. *Argon lasers:* Well absorbed by pigmented bacteria.
   - Used for depigmentation, incision/excision of hemorrhagic lesions, hemostasis.
   - Lethal to black pigmented bacteria, curing of composite materials, tooth whitening, intraoral soft tissue surgery.
2. *Diode lasers:* No interaction with hard tissues.
   a. FDA approved for sulcular debridement and oral soft tissue surgery.
   b. Used for caries and calculus detection, treatment of dentin hypersensitivity, pulpotomy, root canal disinfection, aphthous ulcer treatment, removal of gingival melanin pigmentation.
3. *Nd: YAG laser:* Better absorption in water (60 mm).
   a. Well absorbed by melanin, Hb, chromatophores—useful in killing in pigmented bacteria.
   b. FDA approved for soft tissue removal, caries removal and sulcular debridement.
   c. Indicated in analgesia, treatment of dentin hypersensitivity, pulpotomy, root canal disinfection, removal of enamel caries, aphthous ulcer treatment, removal of gingival melanin pigmentation.
4. *Erbium lasers:* These have emerged as promising laser systems for periodontal infections.
   a. FDA approved for caries removal and cavity preparation, soft tissue surgery, sulcular debridement and osseous surgery.
   b. Caries removal and cavity preparation, modification of enamel and dentin surfaces.

Note: *During CO_2 and erbium laser irradiation, caution should be taken not to contact enamel surface as it might cause melting.*

Low Level Laser Therapy (LLLT)

Therapeutic lasers/cold lasers. Improved healing, decreased pain and swelling.

Doses of LLLT: Gingiva = 2–3 J/cm^2, teeth and bone = 2–4 J/cm^2

Applications: Hypersensitivity, postsurgical cases, herpes labialis, trigeminal neuralgia, aphthous ulcers, periodontitis.

Advantages of Lasers

Better Hemostasis, minimal wound contraction and bactericidal effect.

Disadvantages and Precautions in Clinical use of Lasers

1. Caution before and during irradiation: Use of glasses for eye protection (patient, operator, and assistants)
   a. Inadvertent irradiation (action in noncontact mode)
   b. Protection of patients eyes, throat, and oral tissues outside the target site
   c. Reflection from shiny metal surfaces
   d. Adequate high speed evacuation to capture the laser plume
2. Risk of excessive tissue destruction by direct ablation and thermal side-effects:

   Destruction of the attachment apparatus at the bottom of pockets.

   Excessive ablation of root surface and gingival tissue within periodontal pockets.

   Thermal injury to the root surface, gingival tissue, pulp and bone tissue.

Clinical Note

Laser-assisted new attachment procedure (LANAP) was introduced by Dr. Robert Gregg and Delwin McCarthy in 1989. The indications for LANAP are periodontal pocket depth (PD) ≥ 4 mm, radiographic evidence of bone loss, and positive laboratory test for presence of putative periodontal pathogens.

Laser Assisted Gingivoplasty (Fig. 19.1a to e)

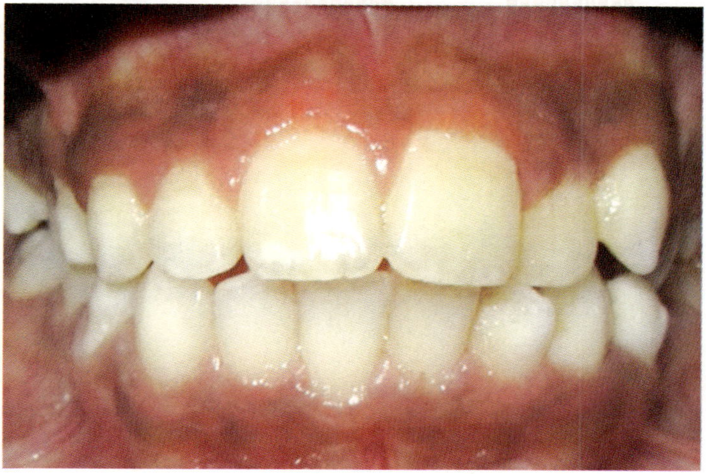

Fig. 19.1a: Preoperative frontal view

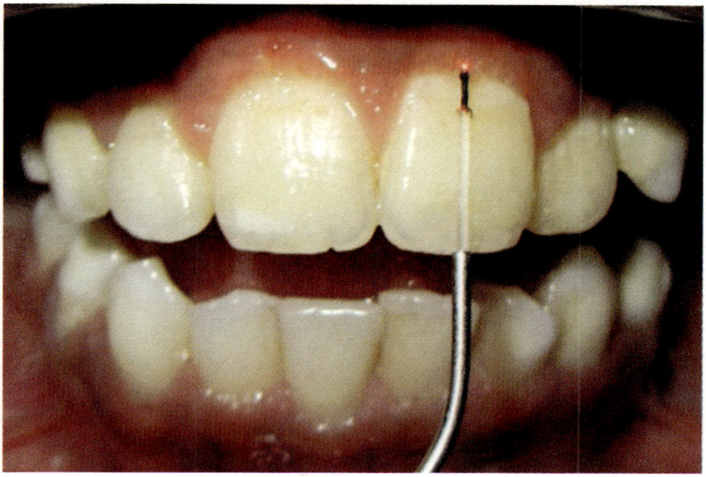

Fig. 19.1b: Diode laser

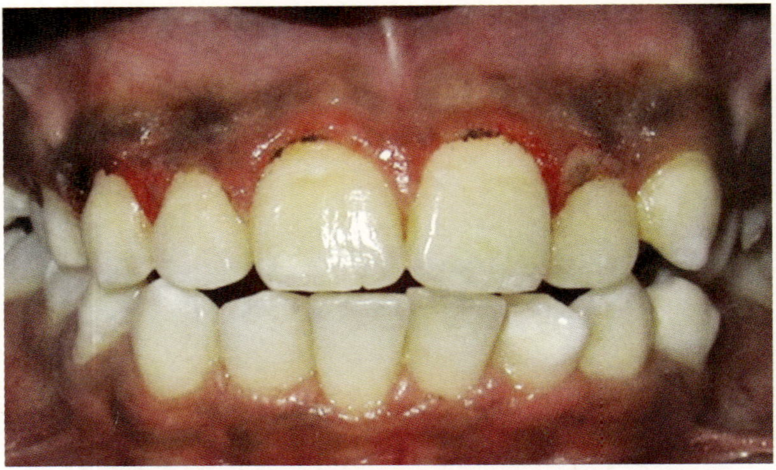

Fig. 19.1c: Immediate postoperative

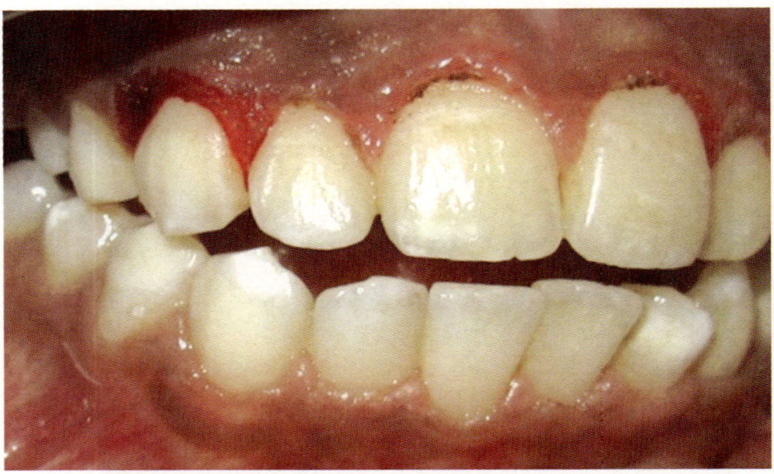

Fig. 19.1d: Right lateral view

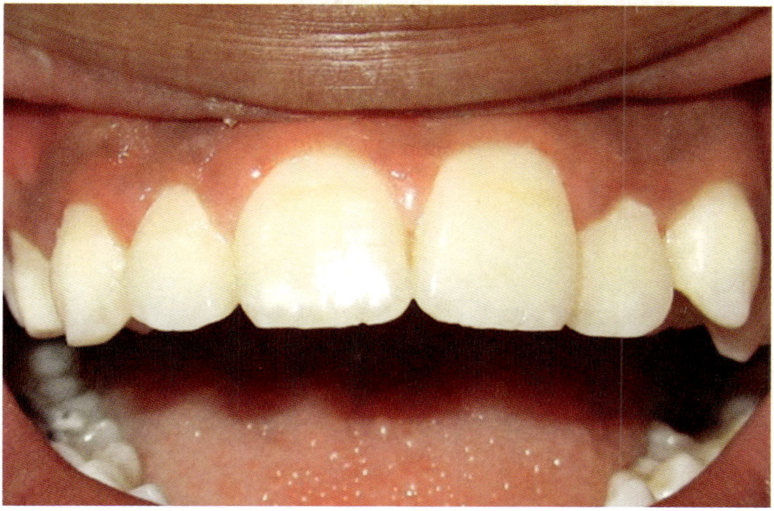

Fig. 19.1e: Postoperative 1 month

Index